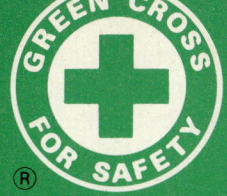 **National Safety Council**

First Aid and CPR

Second Edition

Level 1

Copyright © 1993, 1991 by Jones and Bartlett Publishers, Inc. All rights reserved. No part of the material protected by this copyright notice may be reproduced or utilized in any form, electronic or mechanical, including photocopying, recording, or by any information storage and retrieval system, without written permission from the copyright owner.

The first aid and CPR procedures in this book are based on the most current recommendations of responsible medical sources. The National Safety Council and the publisher, however, make no guarantee as to, and assume no responsibility for, the correctness, sufficiency or completeness of such information or recommendations. Other or additional safety measures may be required under particular circumstances.

Library of Congress Cataloging-in-Publication Data

First aid and CPR. Level 1/National Safety Council—2nd ed.
   p. cm.
   Includes bibliographical references and index.
   ISBN 0-86720-792-2
   1. First aid in illness and injury. 2. CPR (First aid) I. National SafetyCouncil.
RC86.7.F558   1993
616.02'52—dc20
                                                  93-221430
                                                      CIP

Vice President and Publisher ■ Clayton E. Jones

Director of Production ■ Paula Carroll
Design and Production ■ PC&F, Inc.
Cover Design ■ Hannus Design Associates

Principal Photographer ■ Rick Nye
Illustrations ■ Chris Young, artist
Greg Kyle, Larry Hall, Matt Hall, illustrators
Other full-color illustrations ■
   Bruce Argyle, M.D.
   H.B. Bectal, M.D.
   Michael D. Ellis
   Murray P. Hamlet, D.V.M.
   Axel W. Hoke, M.D.
   Sherman A. Minton, M.D.
   Eugene Robertson, M.D.
   Richard C. Ruffalo, D.M.D.
   Jeffrey Saffle, M.D.
   Clifford C. Snyder, M.D.
   Charles E. Stewart, M.D.
   Health Edco

Jones and Bartlett Publishers
One Exeter Plaza
Boston, MA 02116
617-859-3900

Printed in the United States of America
10 9 8 7 6 5

Welcome Message

Congratulations on your decision to take National Safety Council first aid training. More than 140,000 Americans die every year from injuries, and one in three suffers a nonfatal injury, so it is likely that at some time in your life you will encounter an emergency requiring first aid.

Your training in what to do and how to do it may help keep someone alive or prevent a more serious injury. Emergencies can happen anywhere and at any time.

We hope you will enjoy learning more about first aid through the careful study and application of the concepts being taught. Your training can make it possible for you to act confidently if someone needs help when seconds count.

It is wonderful to be able to save a life or aid someone who has been injured! Protecting life and promoting health have been the Council's only mission since 1913.

On behalf of the National Safety Council, as well as our local safety councils and training agencies, I wish you success in your first aid training program.

Sincerely,

Gerard F. Scannell

Gerard F. Scannell, President
National Safety Council

Table of Contents

Chapter 1: Introduction — 1
Chapter 2: Victim Assessment — 3
Chapter 3: Basic Life Support — 7
Chapter 4: Shock — 26
Chapter 5: Bleeding and Wounds — 31
Chapter 6: Specific Body Area Injuries — 35
Chapter 7: Poisoning — 47
Chapter 8: Burns — 58
Chapter 9: Cold- and Heat-Related Injuries — 65
Chapter 10: Bone, Joint, and Muscle Injuries — 71
Chapter 11: Medical Emergencies — 77
Chapter 12: First Aid Skills — 83
Chapter 13: Moving and Rescuing Victims — 89
Index — 92

1 Introduction

The Size of the Injury Problem

Injuries are one of the most serious public health problems. Injuries are the leading cause of death and disability in children and young adults. They destroy the health, lives, and livelihoods of millions of people.

- Each year, more than 140,000 Americans die from injuries (including accidents, suicides, and homicides), and one person in three suffers a nonfatal injury.
- Preceded by heart disease, cancer, and stroke, injury is the fourth leading cause of death among all Americans.
- One of every eight hospital beds is occupied by an injured patient.
- Every year, more than 80,000 Americans suffer unnecessary but permanently disabling injuries of the brain or spinal cord.
- Injury is the leading reason for physician contacts. And more than 25% of hospital emergency room visits are for the treatment of injuries.

Need for First Aid Training

Because of the size and magnitude of the injury problem, everyone must expect sooner or later to be present when an injury or sudden illness strikes. The outcome of such misfortune frequently depends not only on the severity of the injury or illness, but on the first aid rendered. Therefore, every person should be trained in first aid.

First aid is the immediate care given to the injured or suddenly ill person. First aid does *not* take the place of proper medical treatment. It consists only of furnishing temporary assistance until competent medical care, *if needed*, is obtained, or until the chance for recovery without medical care is assured. **Most injuries and illnesses require only first aid care.**

Properly applied, first aid may mean the difference between life and death, rapid recovery and long hospitalization, or temporary disability and permanent injury.

Percentages of years of potential life lost to injury, cancer, heart disease, and other diseases before age 65. Modified from Centers for Disease Control.

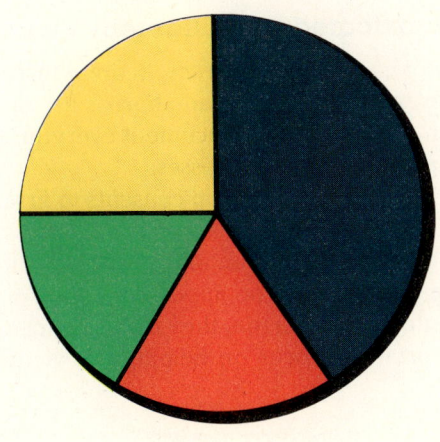

- Heart Disease, 16.4%
- Cancers, 18.0%
- Injury, 40.8%
- All other diseases, 24.8%

Legal Aspects of First Aid

Duty to Act

No one is required to render aid when no legal duty to do so exists. For example, even a physician could ignore a stranger suffering a heart attack or a fractured bone. Moral obligations exist, but they may not be the same as a legal obligation to give aid.

Duty to act may occur in the following situations:

1. **When employment requires it.** If your employment has designated you to render first aid and you are called to an accident scene, then you have a duty to act. Examples include law enforcement officers, park rangers, lifeguards, and teachers who have a job description usually designating the giving of first aid.

2. When a preexisting responsibility exists. You may have a preexisting relationship with another person which demands being responsible for them (e.g., parent-child, driver-passenger) although it is not spelled out in your job description. You must give first aid should they need it.

3. After beginning first aid. Once you start first aid, you cannot stop. Duty to give first aid is usually questioned only when a person fails to act.

Standards of Care

Standards of care ensure quality care and protection for injured or suddenly sick victims. The elements making up a standard of care include:

1. The type of rescuer. A first aider should provide the level and type of care expected of a reasonable person with the same amount of training and in similar circumstances.

2. Published recommendations. Emergency care-related organizations and societies publish recommended first aid procedures. For example, the American Heart Association publishes procedures for giving CPR.

Obtain Consent to Help

You should obtain the victim's approval or permission before starting first aid. This permission is known as **consent.**

- When a victim gives permission to a first aider to help, this is known as **actual consent.** Oral or written permission is valid.
- Consent should be obtained from every conscious, mentally competent adult.
- Permission is implied for giving care for an unconscious victim and is known as **implied consent.** A first aider should not hesitate to treat an unconscious victim.
- Consent should be obtained from the parent or guardian of a victim who is a child, or of one who is an adult but is mentally incompetent. If a parent or guardian is not available, emergency first aid to maintain life may be given without consent. Do *not* withhold first aid from a minor just to obtain parental or guardian permission.
- Psychological emergencies present difficult problems of consent. Under most conditions, a police officer is the only person with the authority to restrain and transport a person against the person's will. However, if the victim is not violent, the situation is similar to that for minors.

Abandonment

Abandonment refers to the behavior of a first aider who begins giving care and then leaves the victim before another person arrives to take over. After starting first aid, you must remain with the victim until he or she is under the care of another person with equal or more training, or until the victim refuses treatment or transportation.

The Right to Refuse Care

A difficult problem involves the conscious, rational, adult victim who is suffering from an actual or potential life-threatening injury or illness but who refuses treatment or transportation. In such situations, make every reasonable effort to convince the victim, or anyone who can influence the victim, to accept first aid and/or transportation. When such a victim refuses to consent, do *not* give first aid or transportation. In such cases, document everything on paper, and if possible, have witnesses.

Parent Refusing Permission to Help a Child

Very rarely will a first aider encounter a parent who refuses permission—usually on moral, ethical, or religious grounds—to care for a seriously injured or ill child. If refusal does occur, make every effort to convince the parent about the seriousness of the problem and the necessity of first aid. If you do not succeed, call the police, document everything on paper, and if possible, have witnesses.

The Intoxicated or Belligerent Victim

If an intoxicated or belligerent victim refuses first aid, make every effort to persuade him or her of the need for such care. If refused, document everything in writing; if possible, have witnesses.

If the intoxicated person consents to first aid, take the greatest possible care. Alcohol and drugs may hide signs and symptoms of an injury. Because first aiders may be repulsed by the appearance and/or attitude of the intoxicated person, they may overlook injuries. It's important to focus on helping the victim.

Good Samaritan Laws

First aiders are covered by a Good Samaritan law in some states. The Good Samaritan laws protect only those acting in good faith and without gross negligence or willful misconduct. If first aiders provide care within the scope of their training, lawsuits are rare. However, if a minor injury is worsened by a first aider, litigation is possible.

2
Victim Assessment

Do *not* move the injured or suddenly ill person until you have a clear idea of the injury or illness and have applied first aid. The exception occurs when the victim is exposed to further danger at the accident scene. If the injury is serious, if it occurred in an area where the victim can remain safely, and if emergency medical service (EMS) attention is readily available, it is sometimes best not to attempt to move the person, but to use first aid at the injury scene until the EMS system responds.

When making a victim assessment, a first aider will consider what witnesses to the accident can tell about the accident, what is observed about the victim, and what the victim can tell.

The first aider must not assume that the obvious injuries are the only ones present because less noticeable injuries may also have occurred. Look for the causes of the injury which may provide a clue as to the extent of physical damage.

In all actions taken during the initial survey the first aider should be especially careful not to move the victim any more than necessary to support life. Any unnecessary movement or rough handling should be avoided because it might aggravate undetected fractures or spinal injuries.

In order to provide good first aid, a person should be able to identify a victim's injury or sudden illness and determine its seriousness. To find out what is wrong and how extensive it is, the first aider should follow a systematic approach known as a victim assessment. Often an abbreviated assessment is sufficient.

A victim assessment attempts to:

- Gain the victim's consent
- Gain the victim's confidence
- Identify the victim's problems and determine which of them require immediate first aid
- Get information about the victim that may prove useful later to the EMS responders and attending medical personnel

A victim assessment of either an injured victim or a medically ill victim is divided into two steps:

- Primary survey
- Secondary survey

Primary Survey

The primary survey covers these areas:
- A—Airway open?
- B—Breathing?
- C—Circulation at carotid pulse?
- H—Hemorrhage: severe bleeding?

The primary survey is the first step in assessing a victim. Its purpose is to find and correct life-threatening conditions.

Airway. Ask: Does the victim have an open airway? If the person is talking or is conscious, the airway is open. Refer to page 8 for the correct and detailed procedures.

Breathing. Ask: Is the victim breathing? Conscious victims are breathing. However, note any breathing difficulties or unusual breathing sounds. If the victim is unconscious, keep the airway open and *look* for the chest to rise and fall, *listen* for breathing, and *feel* for air coming out of the victim's nose and mouth. See page 9 for the correct and detailed procedures.

Circulation. Ask: Is the victim's heart beating? Determine this by feeling for a pulse at the side of the neck (carotid pulse). Refer to page 10 for the correct and detailed procedures.

Hemorrhage. Ask: Is the victim severely bleeding? Check for severe bleeding by looking, if necessary, over the victim's entire body for blood-soaked clothing as a sign of severe bleeding. See Chapter 5 for the correct and detailed procedures.

Secondary Survey

Having completed the primary survey and attended to any life-threatening problems it uncovers, take a closer look at the victim and make a systematic assessment called the secondary survey.

Look for important signs and symptoms of injury. A **sign** is something the first aider sees, hears, or feels (e.g., pale face, no respiration, cool skin). A **symptom** is something the victim tells the first aider about (e.g., nausea, back pain, no sensation in the extremities).

TABLE 2–4 Victim Assessment

Scene Survey

- dangerous hazards?
- number of victims?
- cause of injury?

Primary Survey (also known as Basic Life Support (BLS))

Check responsiveness/protect spine
A = Airway open? (head-tilt/chin-lift)
B = Breathing? (look at chest; listen and feel for air)
C = Circulation? (pulse at carotid?)
H = Hemorrhage? (severe bleeding; personal protection)

Secondary Survey

Interview

- Introduce self/reassure/victim's name/obtain consent/ask questions:
    S = Signs/Symptoms (chief complaint)?
        P = Period of pain (how long)?
        A = Area (where)?
        I = Intensity?
        N = Nullify (what stops it)?
    A = Allergies?
    M = Medications currently taking?
    P = Pertinent past medical history?
    L = Last oral intake: solid or liquid? when and how much?
    E = Events leading to injury or illness?

Vital signs

- Pulse: rate?
- Respiration: rate/sounds?
- Skin condition: temperature/color/moisture?
- Capillary refill?

Head-to-Toe Examination (use **LAF**: L = Look; A = Ask; F = Feel)

Head:	■ Bleeding/deformity/CSF (ears/nose)/mouth clear/cyanosis?
Eyes:	■ Pupils: equal & react to light (PEARL)/inner eyelid color?
Chest:	■ Wounds/penetrating object? ■ Pain (with/without rib spring)?
Abdomen:	■ Wounds/penetrating object? ■ Pain/guarding/rigidity (with/without gentle pushing)?
Extremities:	■ Wounds/deformity/tenderness (compare 2 sides)? ■ pulses? ■ capillary refill?
Spinal cord:	■ Finger/toe wiggle? ■ Touch finger/toe for sensation? ■ Hand squeeze/foot push?

Medical Alert Tag?

The secondary survey is done to discover problems that do not pose an immediate threat to life but may do so if they remain uncorrected. The secondary survey can detect less easily noticed injuries that can be aggravated by mishandling and can find problems which the EMS personnel and other medical authorities might find useful. If a victim with a spinal injury is mishandled, he or she could suffer spinal damage, leading to paralysis. Also, a closed fracture can become an open fracture if not immobilized.

The secondary survey is a head-to-toe examination. Start by examining the victim's head, then neck, trunk, and extremities, looking for abnormalities such as swelling, discoloration, and tenderness, which might indicate an unseen injury. (See Table 2.1)

Putting It All Together

The victim assessment will be influenced by whether the victim is suffering from a medical problem or an injury, whether the victim is conscious or unconscious, and whether life-threatening conditions are present. Remember to first conduct a primary survey and correct any problems it uncovers before going on to the secondary survey.

Medical Alert Tag

A medical alert emblem tag worn as a necklace or as a bracelet attracts attention in an emergency situation. These tags contain the wearer's medical problem and a 24-hour telephone number to call in case of an emergency. Do *not* remove a medical alert tag from an injured or sick person.

Calling the Emergency Medical Services (EMS) System for Help*

In many communities, to receive emergency assistance of every kind you just dial 9–1–1. Check to see if this is true in your community. An emergency number should be listed on the inside cover of your telephone directory.

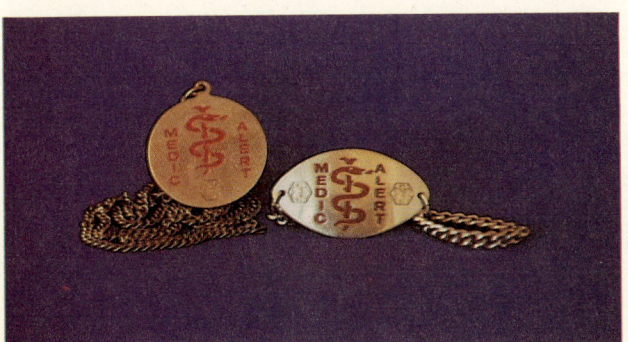

Medical alert tag

To receive the best emergency medical help fast, you should keep a list of phone numbers for the following services near your telephone.

1. ***The rescue squad.*** Often part of the local fire department, these specially trained paramedics are likely to respond swiftly and competently.

2. ***The police.*** They may or may not be able to respond with medically trained personnel; however, they can get someone to the hospital quickly.

3. ***Ambulance service.*** Some services have trained paramedics; others do not.

4. ***Your doctor.*** Your own doctor may not be available, but he or she should be alerted if an emergency has occurred.

5. ***Poison control center.*** In some communities, this service will give information to doctors only. Call before an emergency occurs to find out.

Give the following information over the phone:

1. ***The victim's location.*** Give city or town, street name, and street number. Give names of intersecting streets or roads and other landmarks if possible. Describe the building. The victim's location may be the single most important information you can provide.

2. ***Your phone number.*** This information is required not only to help prevent false calls but, more importantly, to allow the center to call back for additional information.

3. ***What has happened.*** Tell the nature of the emergency (traffic accident, heart attack, dog bite, and so on).

4. ***Number of persons needing help and any special conditions.*** Tell the number of people involved. Tell about any special problems, such as several flights of stairs and no elevators, or the presence of a guard dog.

5. ***Condition of the victim(s).*** Tell about such things as no breathing or pulse, severe bleeding, unconsciousness.

6. ***What is being done for the victim(s).*** Tell about CPR, how the bleeding is being controlled, and so on.

Always be the last to hang up the phone. The EMS system dispatcher may need to ask more questions about how to find you. They may also tell you what to do until help arrives.

Speak slowly and clearly. Shouting is difficult to understand.

According to the National Emergency Number Association, 75 percent of the population and 25 percent of the geographic area in the United States have 9-1-1 coverage. Record your local community emergency telephone numbers and other information on this book's back cover.

SKILL SCAN: Primary Survey

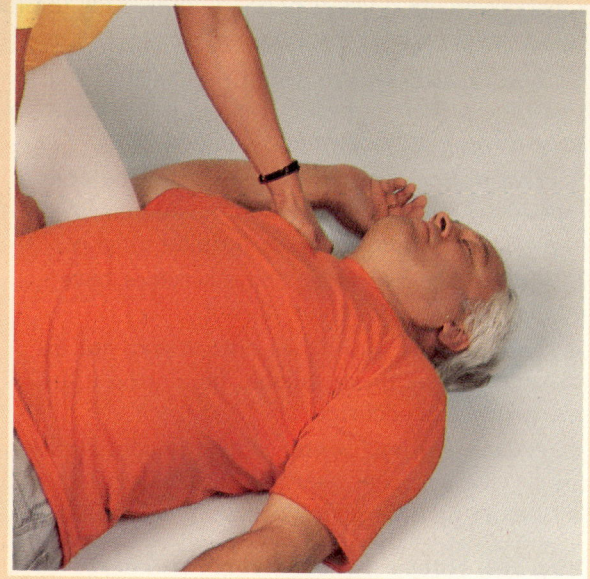

Responsive?

A = Airway open?

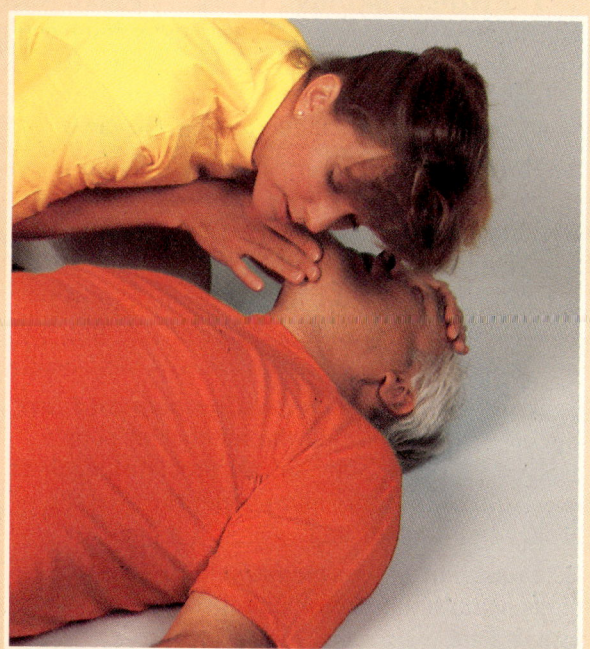

B = Breathing?

C = Circulation at carotid pulse?

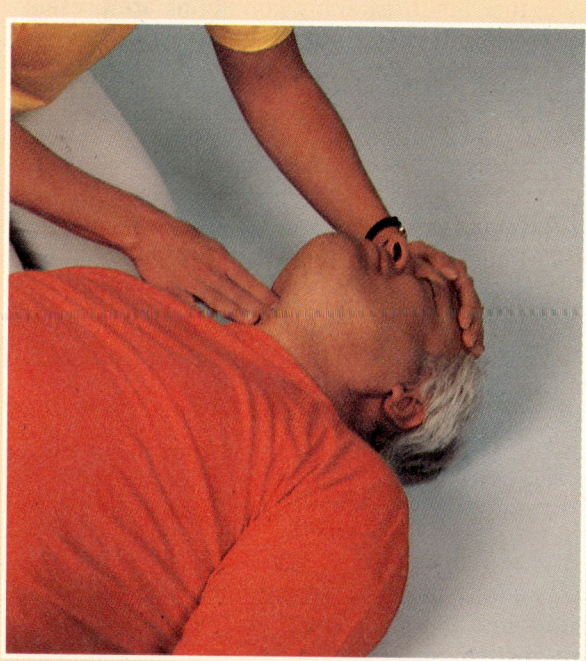

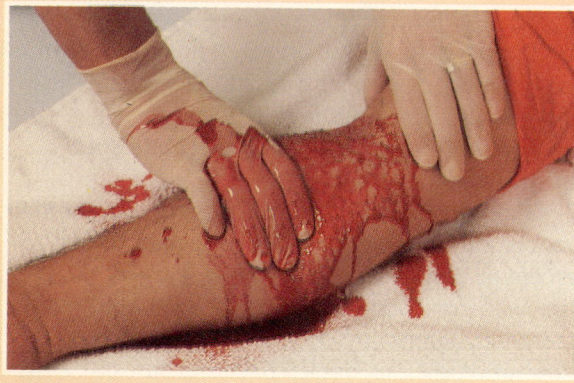

H = Hemorrhage—severe bleeding?

3
Basic Life Support*

What is CPR?

Cardiopulmonary resuscitation (CPR) combines rescue breathing (also known as mouth-to-mouth breathing) and external chest compressions. *Cardio* refers to the heart and *pulmonary* refers to the lungs. *Resuscitation* refers to revive. Proper and prompt CPR serves as a holding action by providing oxygen to the brain and heart until advanced cardiac life support (ACLS) can be provided.

Need for CPR Training

Heart disease causes more than half the deaths in North America. About two-thirds of these deaths are from heart attacks, and more than half of these were dead on arrival (DOA) at a hospital. Sudden death related to heart attacks is the most prominent medical emergency in the United States today.

It is possible that a large number of these deaths could be prevented by prompt action to provide rapid entry into the EMS system, prompt CPR, and early defibrillation. CPR can save heart attack victims, and it can also save lives in cases of drowning, suffocation, electrocution, and drug overdose. Use CPR any time a victim's breathing and heart have stopped. Use rescue breathing whenever there is a pulse but no breathing.

When to Start CPR

Trained people need to be able to:
- Recognize the signs of cardiac arrest
- Provide CPR, and
- Call for the emergency medical services (EMS).

Most people suffering a fatal heart attack die within two hours of the first signs and symptoms of the attack.

Activate the EMS system and start CPR as soon as possible! Victims have a good chance of surviving if:
- CPR is started within the first four minutes of heart stoppage, and
- They receive advanced cardiac life support within the next four minutes.

Brain damage begins after four to six minutes and is certain after ten minutes when no CPR is given.

Signs of Successful CPR

Successful CPR refers to correct CPR performance, not victim survival. Even with successful CPR, most victims will not survive unless they receive advanced cardiac life support (e.g., defibrillation, oxygen, and drug therapy). CPR serves as a holding action until such medical care can be provided. Early bystander CPR (started in less than four minutes after cardiac arrest) coupled with an EMS system with advanced cardiac life support capability (within eight minutes) can increase survival chances to more than 40 percent.

Check CPR's effectiveness by:
- Watching chest rise and fall with each rescue breath

*Based on the 1992 American Heart Association, Guidelines for Cardiopulmonary Resuscitation and Emergency Cardiac Care, JAMA, 1992; 268:2172

TABLE 3-1 Chances of Survival (Survival Rate %)

		Time Until Advanced Cardiac Life Support Begins		
		<8 min.	8-16 min.	>16 min.
Time Until Basic Life Support (CPR)	<4 min.	43%	19%	10%
	4-8 min.	27%	19%	6%
	>8 min.	N/A	7%	0%

Source: National Ski Patrol, based upon Eisenberg, et. al., JAMA, 1979; 241:1905–1907.

- Checking pulse after first minute of CPR and every few minutes afterward to determine if a pulse has returned.
- Having a second rescuer feel for carotid pulse while giving chest compressions. A pulse should be felt each time a compression is made. If alone, do not try to give compressions with one hand while checking for a pulse at the same time.

When to Stop CPR

Stop resuscitation efforts when any of the following occurs:

- Victim revives (regains pulse and breathing). Though hoped for, most victims also require advanced cardiac procedures before they regain their heart and lung functions.
- Replaced by either another trained rescuer or EMS system
- Too exhausted to continue
- Scene becomes unsafe
- A physician tells you to stop
- Cardiac arrest lasts longer than 30 minutes (with or without CPR). This suggestion is controversial, but is supported by the National Association of Emergency Medical Services Physicians.

Recovery Position

For an unconscious, breathing, uninjured victim, use the *recovery position*:

- Roll victim onto side (if no evidence of head or neck injury)
- Place hand of upper arm under chin to support it
- Flex leg to prevent rolling

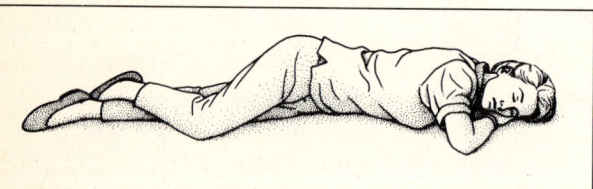

What about the Victim's Clothing?

Usually it's not necessary to remove or loosen victim's clothing. Remove or loosen clothing if:

- Collar does not allow feeling carotid pulse;
- Heavy clothing does not allow locating the notch at the sternum's tip
- Unable to find correct hand position
- Your locale allows EMS personnel to remove by cutting, ripping, or pulling up a victim's clothing in order to bare the chest. This includes either cutting a woman's bra or slipping it up to her neck.

How Does CPR Work?

Chest compressions and/or direct heart compressions create enough pressure within the chest cavity to cause blood to move through the heart and circulatory system. Effective chest compressions provide only one-fourth to one-third of normal blood flow. Rescue breaths provide 16 percent oxygen content—enough to sustain life.

When *NOT* to Start CPR

Usually start CPR whenever pulselessness occurs. However, do not start CPR if positive signs of death appear:

- Decapitation and/or severe mutilation
- Rigor mortis
- Evidence of tissue decomposition
- Lividity (purple-reddish color showing on parts of body closest to ground)

Do not start CPR if evidence exists that the victim has been in cardiac arrest for more than 30 minutes withour prior resuscitation efforts. Exceptions include cold water drowning victims (National Association of Emergency Medical Physicians' recommendation).

Do not start CPR when "do not resuscitate" orders apply—usually in writing and decided upon by victim's family and physician.

Do not start CPR in an unsafe environment or situation. In such cases and if possible, move the victim to a safe location and then begin CPR.

How Can an Untrained Rescuer Help

An untrained rescuer can help by:

- Going for help
- Checking breathing and pulse following directions from trained rescuer
- Performing CPR following directions from trained rescuer

If trained rescuer is exhausted, an untrained rescuer can give chest compressions while the trained rescuer gives rescue breaths. The trained rescuer can explain what to do. Instructions would include:

- Finding the proper hand position
- Keeping the fingers off victim's chest
- Keeping the arms straight and shoulders over victim's chest

- Performing five chest compressions at proper rate and depth, stopping while trained rescuer gives one breath, then having the untrained rescuer start another cycle with five chest compressions.

If the untrained rescuer adequately performs chest compressions, allow him/her to continue helping you.

Dangerous Complications of CPR

Vomiting may occur during CPR. If it happens it is usually before CPR has begun or within the first minute after beginning CPR. Inhaling vomit (aspiration) into the lungs can produce a type of pneumonia that can kill even after successful rescue efforts.

In case of vomiting:

1. Turn victim onto his/her side and keep there until vomiting ends.
2. Wipe vomit out of victim's mouth with your fingers wrapped in a cloth.
3. Reposition victim onto his/her back and resume rescue breathing/CPR if needed.

Stomach (gastric) distention describes stomach bulging from air. It is especially common in children.

- Caused by:
  1. Rescue breaths given too fast
  2. Rescue breaths given too forcefully
  3. Partially or completely blocked airway
- Dangerous because:
  1. Air in stomach pushes against lungs, making it difficult or impossible to give full breaths
  2. Possibility of inhaling vomit into the lungs
- Prevent or minimize by:
  1. Trying to blow just hard enough to make chest rise
  2. Keeping the airway open during inhalations and exhalations
  3. Using mouth-to-nose method
  4. Slow rescue breathing—one-and-a-half to two seconds each—pause between breaths so you can take another breath
  5. Retilting head to open airway

Inhalation of foreign substances (known as aspiration). Foreign substances have no place in the lungs. Three types of substances can create potentially life-threatening situations:

- Particulate matter aspiration—can stop-up airway
- Nongastric liquid aspiration—mainly due to fresh- and salt-water drowning
- Gastric acid aspiration—effects of gastric acid on lung tissue can be equated with a chemical burn.

Help prevent vomiting by placing victim on his/her left side. This position keeps the stomach from spilling its contents into esophagus by keeping the bottom end of esophagus (located where it enters the stomach) above the stomach.

Chest compression-related injuries can happen even with proper compressions. Injuries may include: rib fractures, rib separation, air and/or blood in chest cavity, bruised lung, lacerations of the lung, liver, or spleen.

Prevent or minimize by:

- Using proper hand location on chest—if too low the sternum's tip can cut into liver
- Keeping fingers off victim's ribs by interlocking fingers
- Pressing straight down instead of sideways
- Giving smooth, regular, and uninterrupted (except when breathing) compressions. Avoid sudden, jerking, jabbing, or stabbing compressions.
- Avoiding pressing chest too deeply

Dentures, loose or broken teeth, or dental appliances. Leave tight-fitting dentures in place to support victim's mouth during rescue breathing. Remove loose or broken teeth, dentures, and/or dental appliances.

Foreign Body Airway Obstruction (Choking)

The National Safety Council reports more than 3,000 choking deaths yearly.

How to Recognize Choking

Partial air exchange:

- Good—indicated by coughing forcefully by a conscious victim.
- Poor—indicated by weak, ineffective cough; high pitched noise; blue, gray, or ashen skin.

Breathing sounds which may indicate partial air exchange:

1. Snoring—tongue may be blocking airway
2. Crowing—voice box spasm
3. Wheezing—airway swelling or spasm
4. Gurgling—blood, vomit, or other liquid in airway

Complete blockage:

- Unable to speak, breathe, or cough
- Clutches neck with one or both hands (known as the "universal distress signal for choking")

Precautions During CPR Training

- Do not practice mouth-to-mouth resuscitation on a person—practice on a manikin.
- Do not practice chest compressions on a person—practice on a manikin.
- Do not practice abdominal or chest thrusts on a person.
- Follow the Centers of Disease Control manikin cleaning procedures.

Do *not* use a training manikin *if* you have:

- Sores on the hands, lips, or face (such as a cold sore)
- An upper respiratory infection (such as a cold or sore throat)
- Known positive Hepatitis B (HBV)
- Been infected by HIV or have AIDS
- An infection or recent exposure to an infectious source

Clean manikin between each student's use by:

1. Scrubbing the manikin's entire face and inside of mouth vigorously with a four-by-four-inch gauze pad saturated with 70 percent alcohol (isopropanol or ethanol);

2. Placing the wet gauze pad over the manikin's mouth and nose for at least 30 seconds. Allow manikin's face to dry.

During training, students should practice and become familiar with mouth-to-barrier devices.

CPR Performance Mistakes

While giving rescue breathing and chest compressions, try to avoid the following mistakes.

Rescue breathing mistakes:

- Inadequate head tilt
- Failing to pinch nose shut
- Not giving slow breaths
- Failing to watch chest and listen for exhalation
- Failing to maintain tight seal around victim's mouth (and/or nose)

Chest compression mistakes:

- Pivoting at knees instead of hips (rocking motion)
- Wrong compression site
- Bending elbows
- Shoulders not above sternum (arms not vertical)
- Fingers touching chest
- Heel of bottom hand not in line with sternum
- Placing palm rather than the heel of the hand on sternum
- Lifting hands off chest between compressions (bouncing movement)
- Incorrect compression rate and/or ratio
- Jerky or jabbing compressions rather than smooth compressions

Victim Size Differences

Children's sizes vary, even if the same ages. For the purpose of basic life support, an infant is anyone younger than one year, and a child is anyone between one and eight years of age. Those over eight years of age are classified as adults.

Basic Life Support Procedures and Techniques

Adult Rescue Breathing and CPR

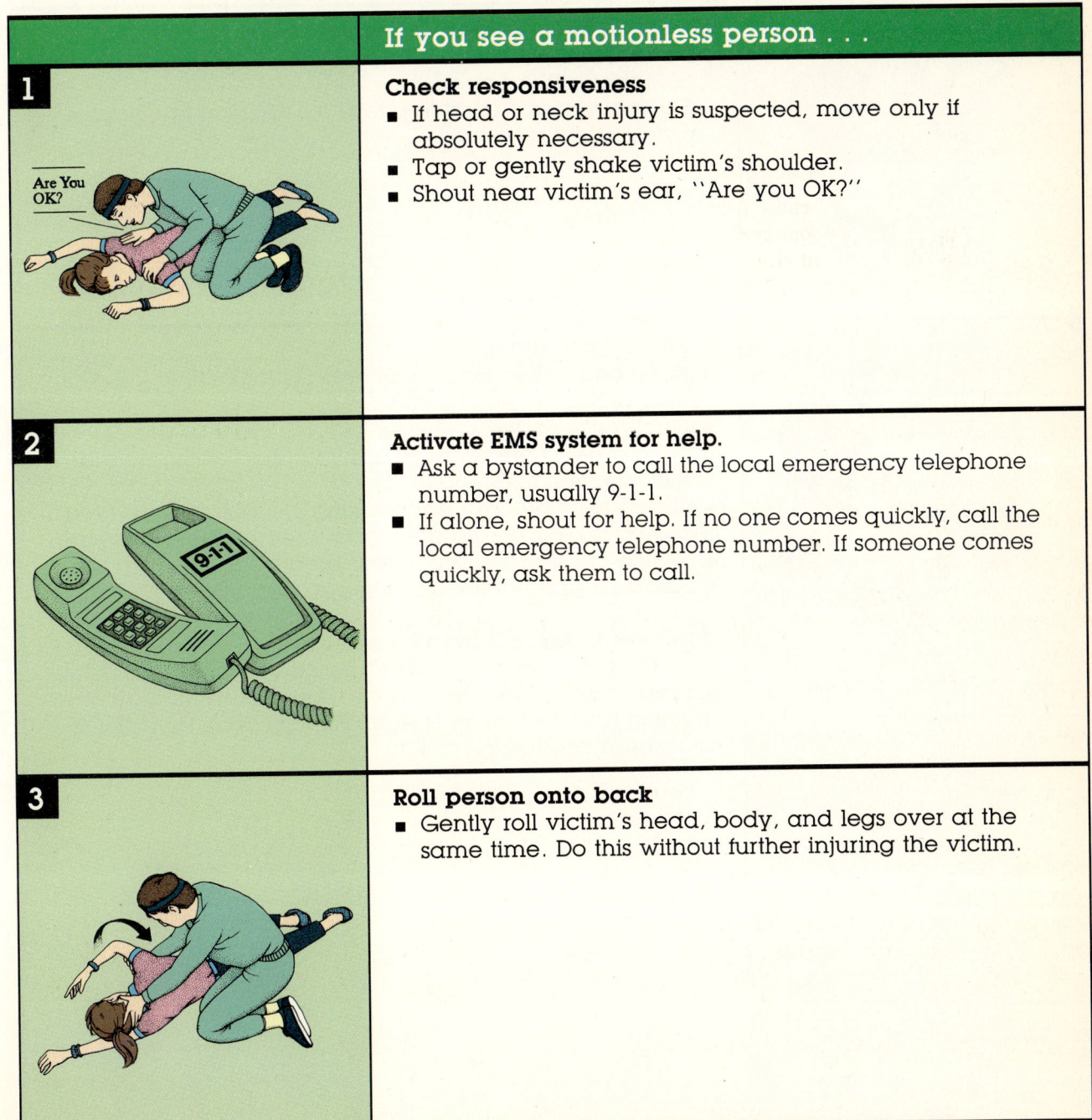

	If you see a motionless person . . .
1	**Check responsiveness** ■ If head or neck injury is suspected, move only if absolutely necessary. ■ Tap or gently shake victim's shoulder. ■ Shout near victim's ear, "Are you OK?"
2	**Activate EMS system for help.** ■ Ask a bystander to call the local emergency telephone number, usually 9-1-1. ■ If alone, shout for help. If no one comes quickly, call the local emergency telephone number. If someone comes quickly, ask them to call.
3	**Roll person onto back** ■ Gently roll victim's head, body, and legs over at the same time. Do this without further injuring the victim.

Adult Rescue Breathing and CPR

4 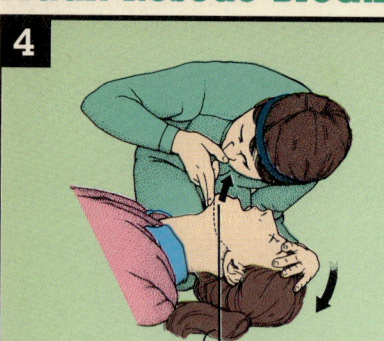	**Open airway** (use head-tilt/chin-lift method) - Place hand nearest infant's head on infant's forehead and apply backward pressure to tilt head back (known as the "sniffing" or neutral position). - Place fingers of other hand under bony part of jaw near chin and lift. Avoid pressing on soft tissues under jaw. - Tilt head backward without closing infant's mouth. - Do not use your thumb to lift the chin. **If you suspect a neck injury** Do not move infant's head or neck. First try lifting chin without tilting head back. If breaths do not go in, slowly and gently bend the head back until breaths can go in.
5 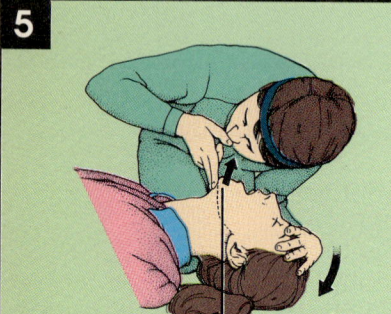	**Check for breathing** (take 3–5 seconds) - Place your ear over victim's mouth and nose while keeping airway open. - *Look* at victim's chest to check for rise and fall; *listen* and *feel* for breathing.
6 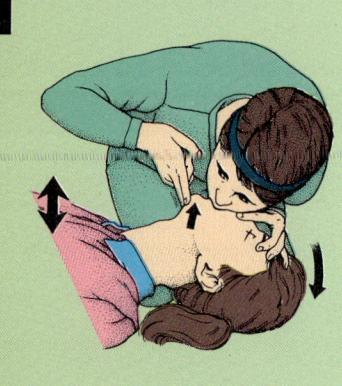	**Give 2 slow breaths** - Keep head tilted back with head-tilt/chin-tilt to keep airway open. - Pinch nose shut. - Take a deep breath and seal your lips tightly around victim's mouth. - Give 2 slow breaths, each lasting 1½ to 2 seconds (you should take a breath after each breath given to victim). - Watch chest rise to see if your breaths go in. - Allow for chest deflation after each breath. **If neither of these 2 breaths went in** Retilt the head and try 2 more breaths. If still unsuccessful, suspect choking, also known as foreign body airway obstruction (use *Unconscious Adult Foreign Body Airway Obstruction* procedures).

Adult Rescue Breathing and CPR

7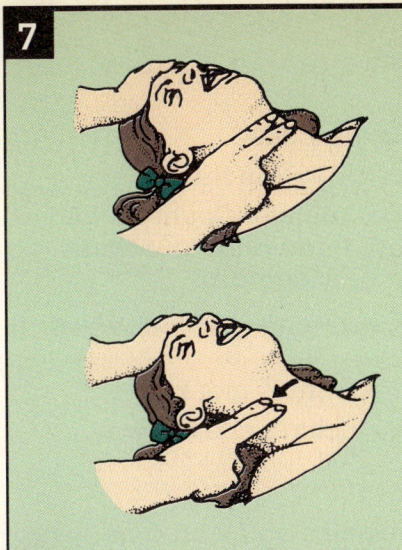

Check for pulse
- Maintain head-tilt with hand nearest head on forehead.
- Locate Adam's apple with 2 or 3 fingers of hand nearest victim's feet.
- Slide your fingers down into groove of neck on side closest to you (do not use your thumb because you may feel your own pulse).
- Feel for carotid pulse (take 5-10 seconds). Carotid artery is used because it lies close to the heart and is accessible.

8

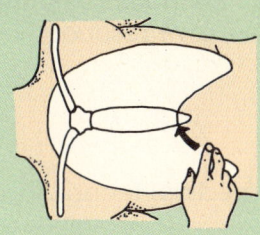

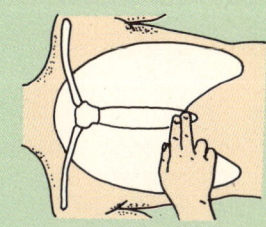

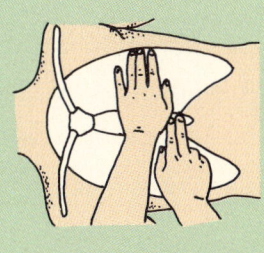

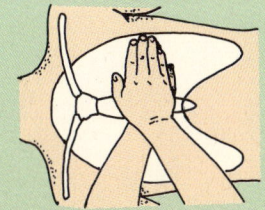

Perform rescue procedures based upon what you found:

If there is a pulse but no breathing
Give one rescue breath (mouth-to-mouth resuscitation) every 5 to 6 seconds. Use the same techniques for rescue breathing found in Step 6 above but only give one. Every minute (10 to 12 breaths) stop and check the pulse to make sure there is a pulse. Continue until:
- Adult starts breathing on his or her own.

OR
- Trained help, such as emergency medical technicians (EMTs), arrive and relieve you.

OR
- You are completely exhausted.

If there is no pulse, give CPR
- Find hand position

   1. Use your fingers to slide up rib cage edge nearest you to notch at the end of sternum.

   2. Place your middle finger on or in the notch and index finger next to it.

   3. Put heel of other hand (one closest to victim's head) on sternum next to index finger.

   4. Remove hand from notch and put it on top of hand on chest.

   5. Interlace, hold, or extend fingers up

Adult Rescue Breathing and CPR

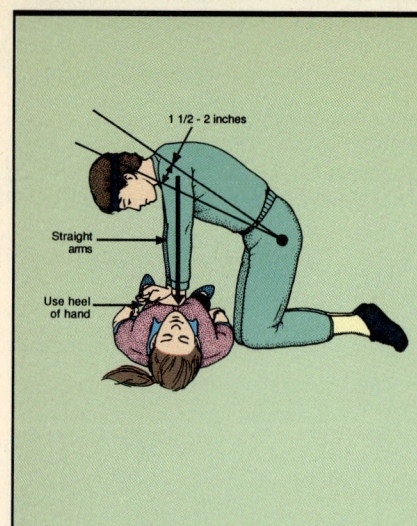

- **Do 15 compressions**
    1. Place your shoulders directly over your hands on the chest.
    2. Keep arms straight and elbows locked.
    3. Push sternum straight down 1½ to 2 inches.
    4. Do 15 compressions at 80 per minute. Count as you push down: "one and, two and, three and, four and, five and, six and, seven and, . . . fifteen and."
    5. Push smoothly; do not jerk or jab; do not stop at the top or at the bottom.
    6. When pushing, bend from your hips, not knees.
    7. Keep fingers pointing across victim's chest, away from you.
- Give 2 slow breaths
- Complete 4 cycles of 15 compressions and 2 breaths (takes about 1 minute) and check the pulse. *If there is no pulse,* restart CPR with chest compressions. Recheck the pulse every few minutes. *If there is a pulse,* give rescue breathing.
- Give CPR or rescue breathing until:
  Victim revives.
  OR
  Trained help, such as emergency medical technicians (EMTs), arrives and relieves you.
  OR
  You are completely exhausted.

Conscious Adult Foreign Body Airway Obstruction (Choking)

	If person is conscious and cannot speak, breathe, or cough . . .
1	**Give up to 5 abdominal thrusts** (Heimlich maneuver): ■ Stand behind the victim. ■ Wrap your arms around victim's waist. (Do not allow your forearms to touch the ribs.) ■ Make a fist with 1 hand and place the thumb side just above victim's navel and well below the tip of the sternum. ■ Grasp fist with your other hand. ■ Press fist into victim's abdomen with 5 quick upward thrusts. ■ Each thrust should be a separate and distinct effort to dislodge the object. After every 5 abdominal thrusts, check the victim and your technique. Note: For advanced pregnant women and obese victims consider using chest thrusts.
2	**Repeat cycles of up to 5 abdominal thrusts until:** ■ Victim coughs up object. OR ■ Victim starts to breathe or coughs forcefully. OR ■ Victim becomes unconscious (activate EMS and start methods for an unconscious victim with finger sweep first). OR ■ You are relieved by EMS or other trained person. Reassess victim and your technique after every 5 thrusts.

Unconscious Adult Foreign Body Airway Obstruction (Choking)

If person is unconscious and breaths have not gone in . . .

1 **Give up to 5 abdominal thrusts** (Heimlich maneuver):
- Straddle victim's thighs.
- Put heel of one hand against middle of victim's abdomen slightly above navel and well below sternum's notch (fingers of hand should point toward victim's head).
- Put other hand directly on top of first hand.
- Press inward and upward using both hands with up to 5 quick abdominal thrusts.
- Each thrust should be distinct and a real attempt made to relieve the airway obstruction. Keep heel of hand in contact with abdomen between abdominal thrusts.

Note: For advanced pregnant women and obese victims consider using chest thrusts.

2 **Perform finger sweep**
- Use only on an unconscious victim. On a conscious victim, it may cause gagging or vomiting.
- Use your thumb and fingers to grasp victim's jaw and tongue and lift upward to pull tongue away from back of throat and away from foreign object.
- If unable to open mouth to perform the tongue-jaw lift, use the crossed-finger method by crossing the index finger and thumb and pushing the teeth apart.
- With index finger of your other hand, slide finger down along the inside of one cheek deeply into mouth and use a hooking action across to other cheek to dislodge foreign object.
- If foreign body comes within reach, grab and remove it. Do not force object deeper.

3 **If the above steps are unsuccessful**
Cycle through the following steps in rapid sequence until the object is expelled or EMS arrives:
- Give 2 rescue breaths. If unsuccessful, retilt head and try 2 more.
- Do up to 5 abdominal thrusts.
- Do a finger sweep.

Adult Basic Life Support Proficiency Checklist

S = self-check / P = partner check / I = instructor check

Adult Rescue Breathing

	S	P	I
1. Check responsiveness	☐	☐	☐
2. Activate EMS	☐	☐	☐
3. Roll victim onto back	☐	☐	☐
4. **A**irway open	☐	☐	☐
5. **B**reathing check	☐	☐	☐
6. 2 slow breaths	☐	☐	☐
7. **C**heck pulse at carotid	☐	☐	☐
8. Rescue breathing (1 every 5 to 6 seconds)	☐	☐	☐
9. Recheck pulse and breathing after first minute, then every few minutes	☐	☐	☐

Adult One-Rescuer CPR

	S	P	I
1. Check responsiveness	☐	☐	☐
2. Activate EMS	☐	☐	☐
3. Roll victim onto back	☐	☐	☐
4. **A**irway open	☐	☐	☐
5. **B**reathing check	☐	☐	☐
6. 2 slow breaths	☐	☐	☐
7. **C**heck pulse at carotid	☐	☐	☐
8. Hand position	☐	☐	☐
9. 15 compressions	☐	☐	☐
10. 2 slow breaths	☐	☐	☐
11. Continue CPR (3 more cycles for total of 4)	☐	☐	☐
12. Recheck pulse	☐	☐	☐
13. Continue CPR (start with compressions)	☐	☐	☐
14. Recheck pulse after first minute, then every few minutes	☐	☐	☐

Conscious Adult Choking Management

	S	P	I
1. Recognize choking	☐	☐	☐
2. Up to 5 abdominal thrusts	☐	☐	☐
3. Reassess	☐	☐	☐
4. Repeat cycles of up to 5 thrusts; reassess after each cycle	☐	☐	☐

Unconscious Adult Choking Management

	S	P	I
1. Check responsiveness	☐	☐	☐
2. Activate EMS	☐	☐	☐
3. Roll victim onto back	☐	☐	☐
4. **A**irway open	☐	☐	☐
5. **B**reathing check	☐	☐	☐
6. Try 2 slow breaths. If unsuccessful, retilt head and try 2 more	☐	☐	☐
7. Up to 5 abdominal thrusts	☐	☐	☐
8. Finger sweep	☐	☐	☐
9. Try 2 slow breaths. If unsuccessful, retilt head and try 2 more	☐	☐	☐
10. Repeat "thrusts, sweep, breaths" sequence	☐	☐	☐

Differences Between Adult and Child (1–8 years) Basic Life Support

IF child . . .	THEN . . .
is **not** responsive	**activate EMS system after 1 minute of resuscitation** (in adults, activate EMS system immediately after determining unresponsiveness)
is **not** breathing, but has a pulse	■ give **1 to 1½ seconds breaths** (in adults give 1½ to 2 seconds breaths) ■ give **1 breath every 3 seconds** (in adults give 1 breath every 5 to 6 seconds)
does **not** have a pulse	■ after locating the tip of the breastbone, lift your fingers off and put heel of the **same hand** on breastbone immediately above where index finger was (adult requires one hand to locate and the other hand placed next to it) ■ give **chest compressions with 1 hand** (nearest feet) while keeping other hand on child's forehead (adult requires 2 hands on victim's chest for compressions) ■ **compress breastbone 1 to 1½ inches** (adults require 1½ to 2 inches) ■ give **one breath after every 5 chest compressions** (one-rescuer adult CPR requires 2 breaths after every 15 compressions)
has a foreign body airway obstruction (choking), and after giving up to 5 abdominal thrusts (Heimlich maneuver), the airway still remains obstructed	look into mouth; **remove foreign body only if seen with finger sweep—do not perform blind finger sweeps** (in an adult, you can perform blind finger sweeps)

Infant (under 1 year) Rescue Breathing and CPR

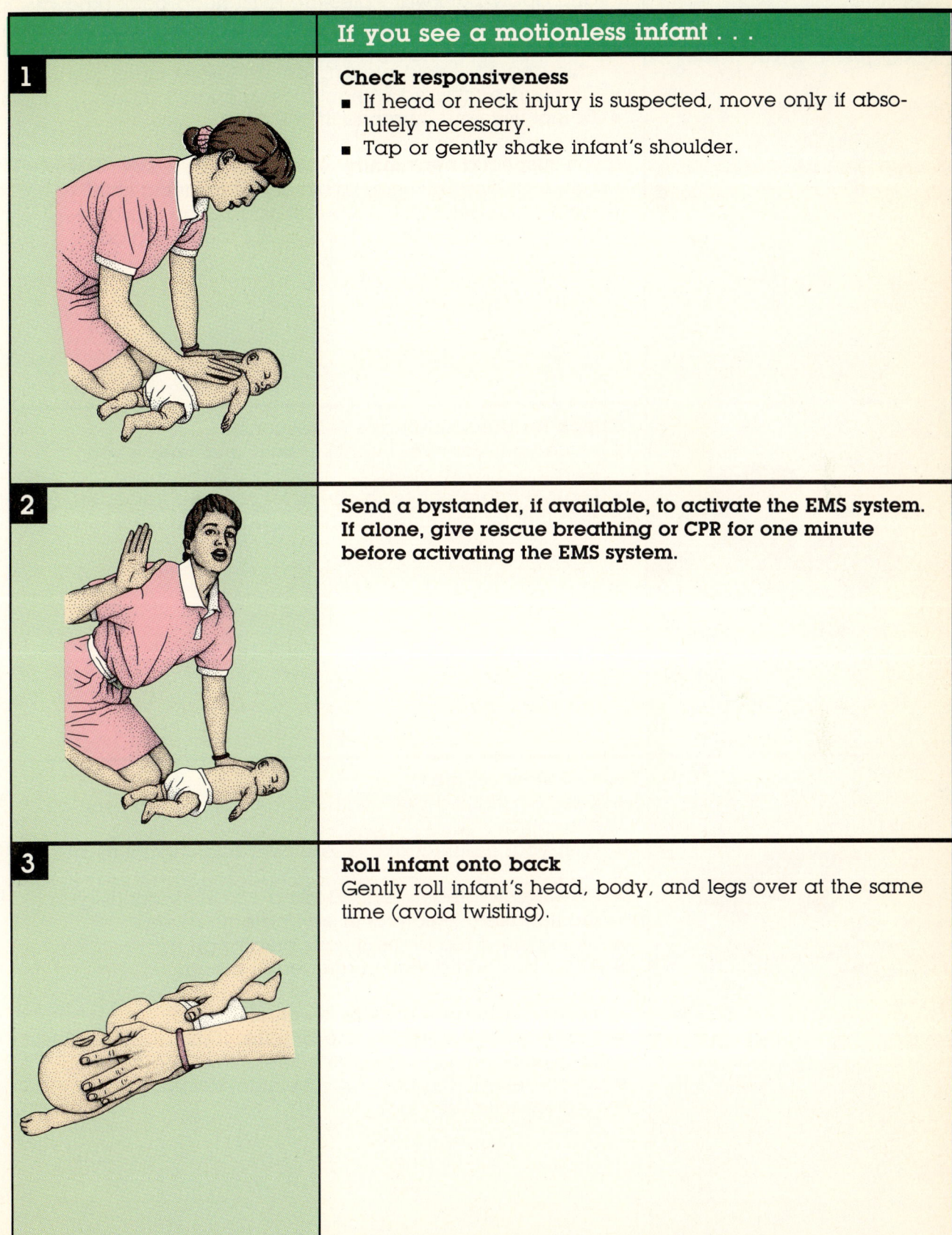

If you see a motionless infant . . .

1. Check responsiveness
- If head or neck injury is suspected, move only if absolutely necessary.
- Tap or gently shake infant's shoulder.

2. Send a bystander, if available, to activate the EMS system. If alone, give rescue breathing or CPR for one minute before activating the EMS system.

3. Roll infant onto back
Gently roll infant's head, body, and legs over at the same time (avoid twisting).

Infant Rescue Breathing and CPR

4

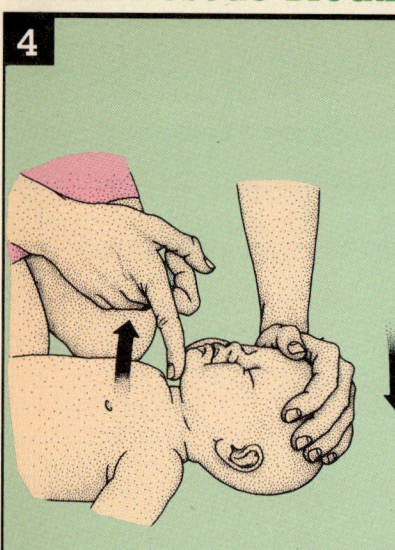

Open airway (use head-tilt/chin-lift method)
- Place hand nearest infant's head on infant's forehead and apply backward pressure to tilt head back (known as the "sniffing" or neutral position).
- Place fingers of other hand under bony part of jaw near chin and lift. Avoid pressing on soft tissues under jaw.
- Tilt head backward without closing infant's mouth.
- Do not use your thumb to lift the chin.

If you suspect a neck injury
Do *not* move victim's head or neck. First try lifting chin without tilting head back. If breaths do not go in, slowly and gently bend the head back until breaths can go in.

5

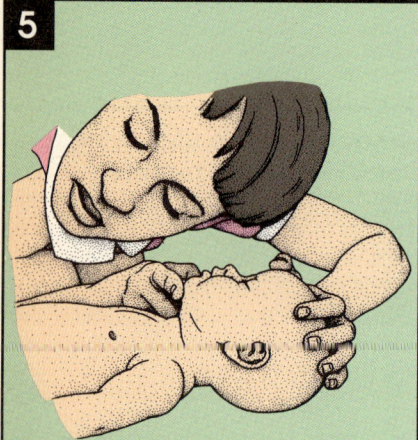

Check for breathing (take 3–5 seconds)
- Place your ear over infant's mouth and nose while keeping airway open.
- Look at infant's chest to check for rise and fall; listen and feel for breathing.

6

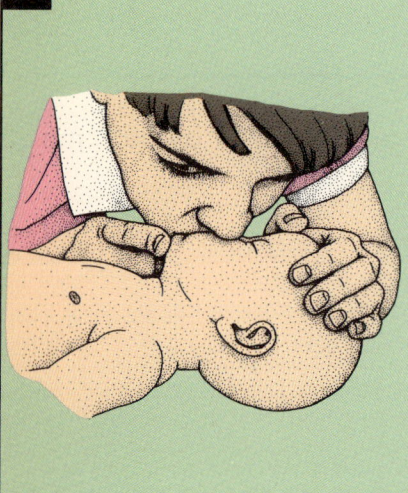

Give 2 slow breaths
- Keep head tilted back with head-tilt/chin-lift to keep airway open
- With your mouth make a seal over infant's mouth and nose.
- Give 2 slow breaths, each lasting 1 to 1½ seconds (you should take a breath after each breath given).
- Watch chest rise to see if your breaths go in.
- Allow for chest deflation after each breath.

If neither of these 2 breaths went in
Retilt the head and try 2 more breaths. If still unsuccessful, suspect choking, also known as foreign body airway obstruction (refer to the Unconscious Infant Foreign Body Airway Obstruction section).

Infant Rescue Breathing and CPR

7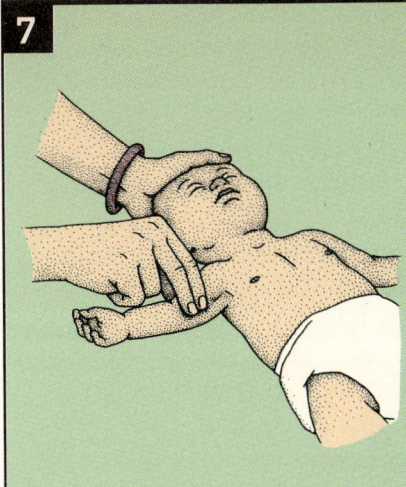

Check for pulse
- Maintain head-tilt with hand nearest head on forehead.
- Feel for pulse located on the inside of the upper arm between the elbow and armpit (known as the brachial).
- Press gently with 2 fingers on inside of arm closest to you.
- Place thumb of same hand on outside of infant's upper arm.

8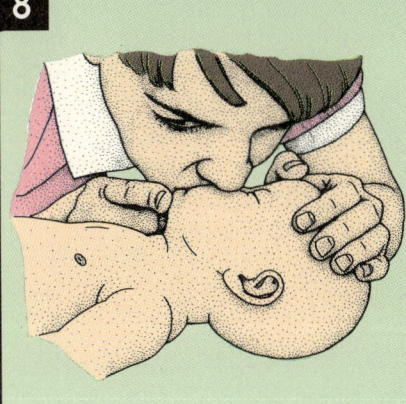

Perform rescue procedures based upon your pulse check

If there is a pulse
Give rescue breaths (mouth-to-mouth resuscitation) every 3 seconds. Use the same techniques for rescue breathing found in Step 6 but only give one breath. Every minute (20 breaths) stop and check the pulse to make sure there is a pulse. Continue until:

- Infant starts breathing on his or her own.

OR

- Trained help, such as emergency medical technicians (EMTs), arrive and relieve you.

OR

- You are completely exhausted.

Infant Rescue Breathing and CPR

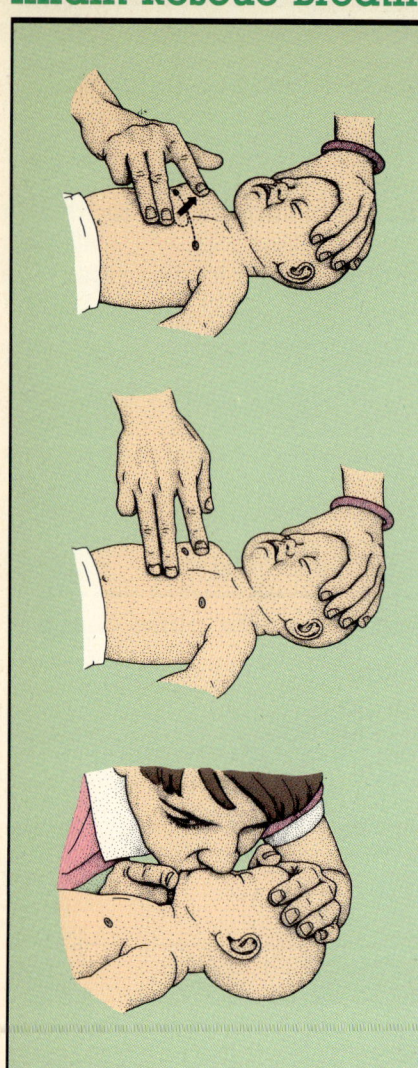

If there is no pulse, give CPR:
- Locate fingers' position
    1. Maintain head-tilt
    2. Imagine a line connecting the nipples
    3. Place 3 fingers on sternum with index finger touching but below imaginary nipple line.
    4. Raise your index finger and use other 2 fingers for compression. If you feel the notch at the end of the sternum, move your fingers up a little.
- Give 5 compressions
    1. Do 5 chest compressions at rate of 100 per minute or count as you push down, "one, two, three, four, five."
    2. Press sternum ½ to 1 inch or about ⅓ to ½ of the depth of the chest.
    3. Keep fingers pointing across the infant's chest away from you. Keep fingers in contact with infant's chest.
    4. Maintain head-tilt with hand nearest head on forehead.
- Give 1 breath
- Complete 20 cycles of 5 compressions and one breath (takes about 1 minute) and check the pulse. If rescuer is alone, activate the EMS system. If there is no pulse, restart CPR with chest compressions. Recheck the pulse every few minutes. If there is a pulse, give rescue breathing.
- Give CPR until:
Infant revives.
OR
Trained help, such as emergency medical technicians (EMTs), arrives and relieves you.
OR
You are completely exhausted.

Conscious Infant Foreign Body Airway Obstruction (Choking)

	If infant is conscious and cannot cough, cry, or breathe...
1	**Give up to 5 back blows** - Hold infant's head and neck with 1 hand by firmly holding infant's jaw between your thumb and fingers. - Lay infant face down over your forearm with head lower than his/her chest. Brace your forearm and infant against your thigh. - Give up to 5 distinct and separate back blows between shoulder blades with the heel of your hand.
2	**Give up to 5 chest thrusts** - Support the back of infant's head. - Sandwich infant between your hands and arms, turn on back, with head lower than his/her chest. Small rescuers may need to support infant on their lap. - Imagine a line connecting infant's nipples. - Place 3 fingers on sternum with your ring finger next to imaginary nipple line on the infant's feet side. - Lift your ring finger off chest. If you feel the notch at the end of the sternum, move your fingers up a little. - Give up to 5 separate and distinct thrusts with index and middle fingers on sternum in a manner similar to CPR chest compressions, but at a slower rate. - Keep fingers in contact with chest between chest thrusts.

3	**Repeat**
	1. Up to 5 back blows
	2. Up to 5 chest thrusts until:
	    - infant becomes unconscious, or
	    - object is expelled and infant begins to breathe or coughs forcefully

Unconscious Infant with Foreign Body Airway Obstruction (Choking)

If infant is motionless . . .

1. Check responsiveness
- If head or neck injury is suspected, move only if absolutely necessary.
- Tap or gently shake infant's shoulder.

2. Send bystander, if available, to activate the EMS system. If alone, resuscitate for one minute before activating the EMS system.

3. Give 2 slow breaths
- Open the airway with head-tilt/chin-lift.
- Seal your mouth over infant's mouth and nose.
- Give 2 slow breaths (1 to 1½ seconds each)

If first 2 breaths do not go in, retilt the head and try 2 more slow breaths.

4. Give up to 5 back blows
- Hold infant's head and neck with 1 hand by firmly holding infant's jaw between your thumb and fingers.
- Lay infant face down over your forearm with head lower than his/her chest. Brace your forearm and infant against your thigh.
- Give up to 5 distinct and separate back blows between shoulder blades with the heel of your hand.

Unconscious Infant with Foreign Body Airway Obstruction (Choking)

5 **Give up to 5 chest thrusts**
- Support the back of infant's head.
- Sandwich infant between your hands and arms, turn on back, with head lower than his/her chest. Small rescuers may need to support infant on their lap.
- Imagine a line connecting infant's nipples.
- Place 3 fingers on sternum with your ring finger next to imaginary nipple line on the infant's feet side.
- Lift your ring finger off chest. If you feel the notch at the end of the sternum, move your fingers up a little.
- Give up to 5 separate and distinct thrusts with index and middle fingers on sternum in a manner similar to CPR chest compressions, but at a slower rate.
- Keep fingers in contact with chest between chest thrusts.

6 **Check mouth for foreign object**
- Grasp both tongue and jaw between your thumb and fingers and lift up.
- If object is seen, remove with a finger sweep by sliding your little finger of the other hand alongside cheek to base of tongue using a hooking action.
- Do not try to remove an unseen object (known as a "blind finger sweep").
- Do not push object deeper.

7 **Repeat**
1. 2 slow breaths (retilt head and try 2 more breaths if first 2 are unsuccessful)
2. Up to 5 back blows
3. Up to 5 chest thrusts
4. Check mouth for foreign object (if object is seen, use finger sweep)

Repeat steps until object is expelled or EMS system arrives. If you are alone and after 1 minute the object has not been expelled then take infant with you and call the EMS system.

4 Shock

Most injuries involve some degree of shock. Shock occurs when the circulatory system fails to deliver oxygenated blood to every part of the body.

Types of Shock

Several types of shock exist; first aiders usually concern themselves mainly with these three types: hypovolemic, fainting, and anaphylactic shock (the latter is better known as a severe allergic reaction).

Hypovolemic

Hypovolemic shock results from blood or fluid loss. If related to blood loss it is best known as hemorrhagic shock.

Signs and Symptoms

- Pale or bluish skin, nailbed, and lips
- Slow capillary filling time
- Cool, wet (clammy) skin; heavy sweating
- Rapid breathing and pulse
- Dilated (enlarged) pupils
- Dull, sunken look to the eyes
- Thirst
- Nausea and vomiting
- Loss of consciousness in severe shock

Even if signs and symptoms have not appeared in a severely injured victim, treat for shock. **First aiders can prevent shock; they cannot reverse it.**

Fainting

Fainting involves a sudden, temporary loss of consciousness. It occurs when the brain's blood flow is interrupted. Numerous causes account for the interrupted blood flow.

Signs and Symptoms

Fainting may occur suddenly or may be preceded by warning signs including any or all of the following:

- Dizziness
- "Seeing spots"
- Nausea
- Paleness
- Sweating

Severe Allergic Reaction (Anaphylactic Shock)

Allergies are usually thought of as causing rashes, itching, or some other short-term discomfort that disappears when the offending agent is removed from contact with the allergic person. There is, however, a more powerful reaction to substances ordinarily eaten or injected called anaphylactic shock, which can occur within minutes and even in some cases within seconds. Such a reaction can cause death if not treated immediately.

The severe allergic response (anaphylactic shock) is triggered by contact with a substance that the individual has previously encountered and the body has identified as an enemy, causing the development of antibodies called IgE. The antibodies, or body defenders, later come in contact with the offending substance and release chemicals (e.g., histamine) that attack the lungs, blood vessels, intestine, and skin. **It is a life-threatening situation!** About 60–80 percent of anaphylactic deaths are caused by an inability to breathe because swollen airway passages obstruct airflow to the lungs. The second most common cause of anaphylactic deaths—about 24 percent—is shock, brought on by insufficient blood circulating through the body.

Signs and Symptoms

One or all of these signs and symptoms may appear:

- Coughing, sneezing, or wheezing
- Difficult breathing
- Tightness and swelling in the throat
- Tightness in the chest
- Severe itching, burning, rash, or hives
- Swollen face, tongue, mouth
- Nausea and vomiting
- Dizziness
- Abdominal cramps
- Blueness (cyanosis) around the lips and mouth
- Unconsciousness

FIRST AID 4: Shock

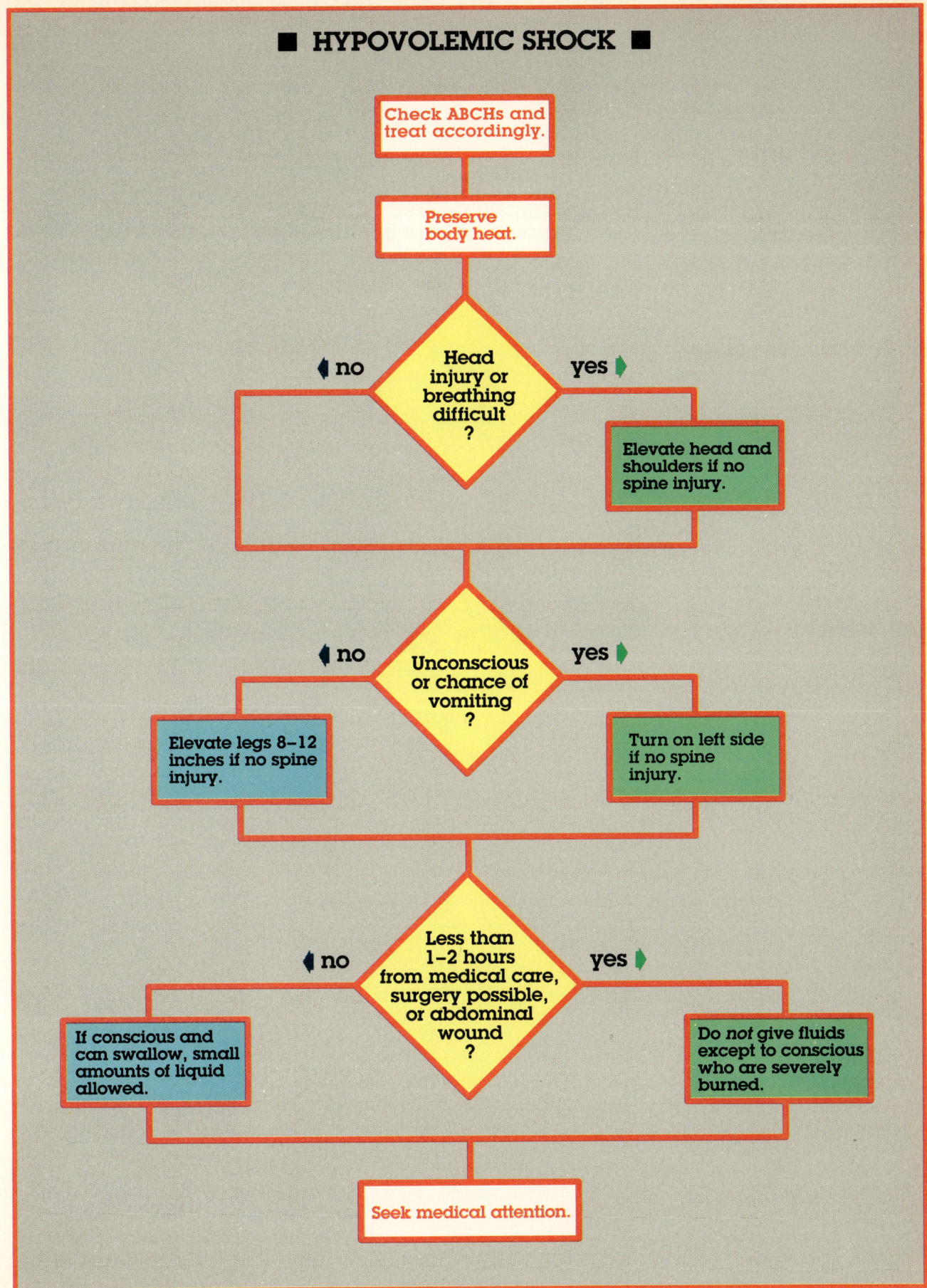

FIRST AID 4: Shock

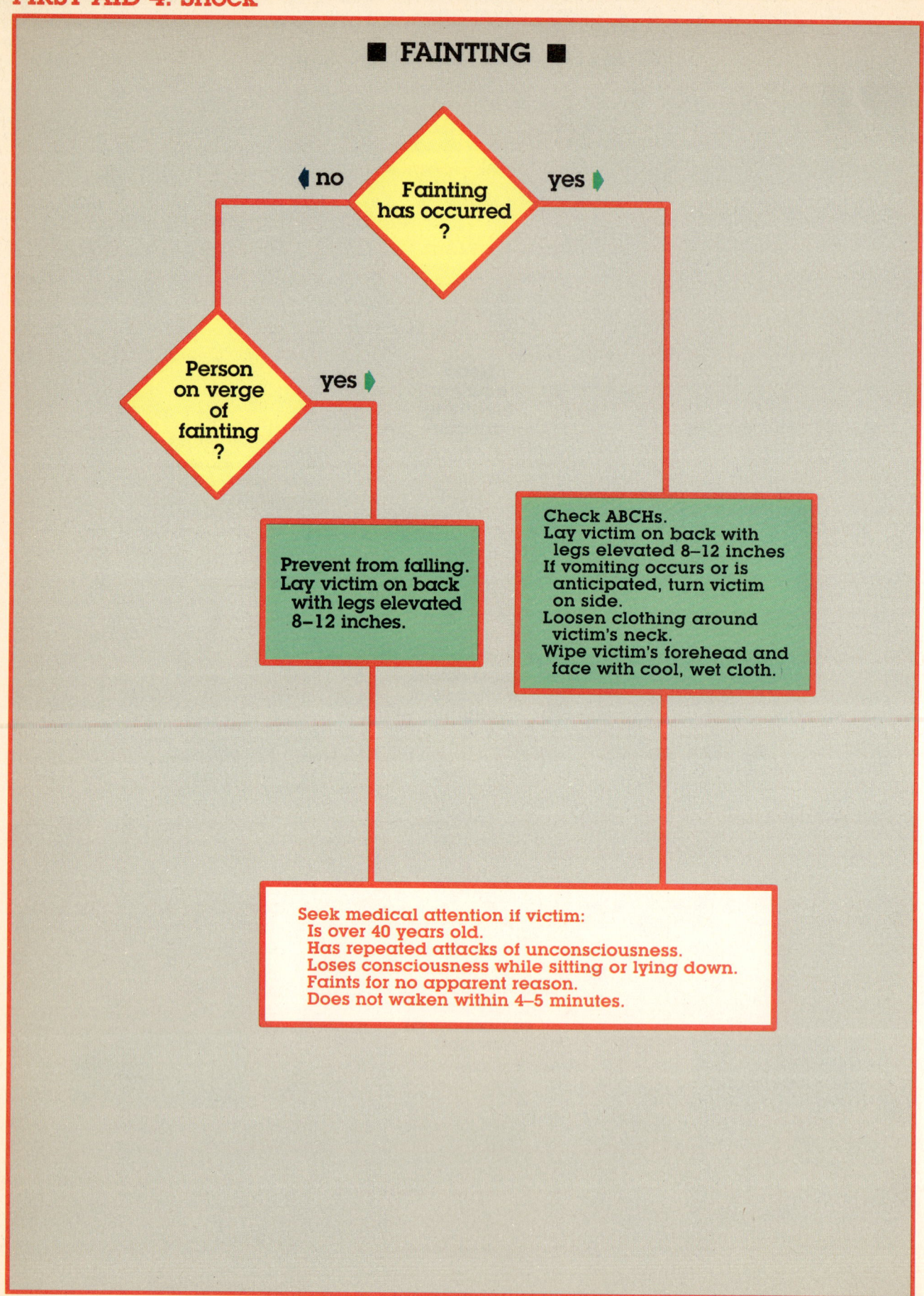

FIRST AID 4: Shock

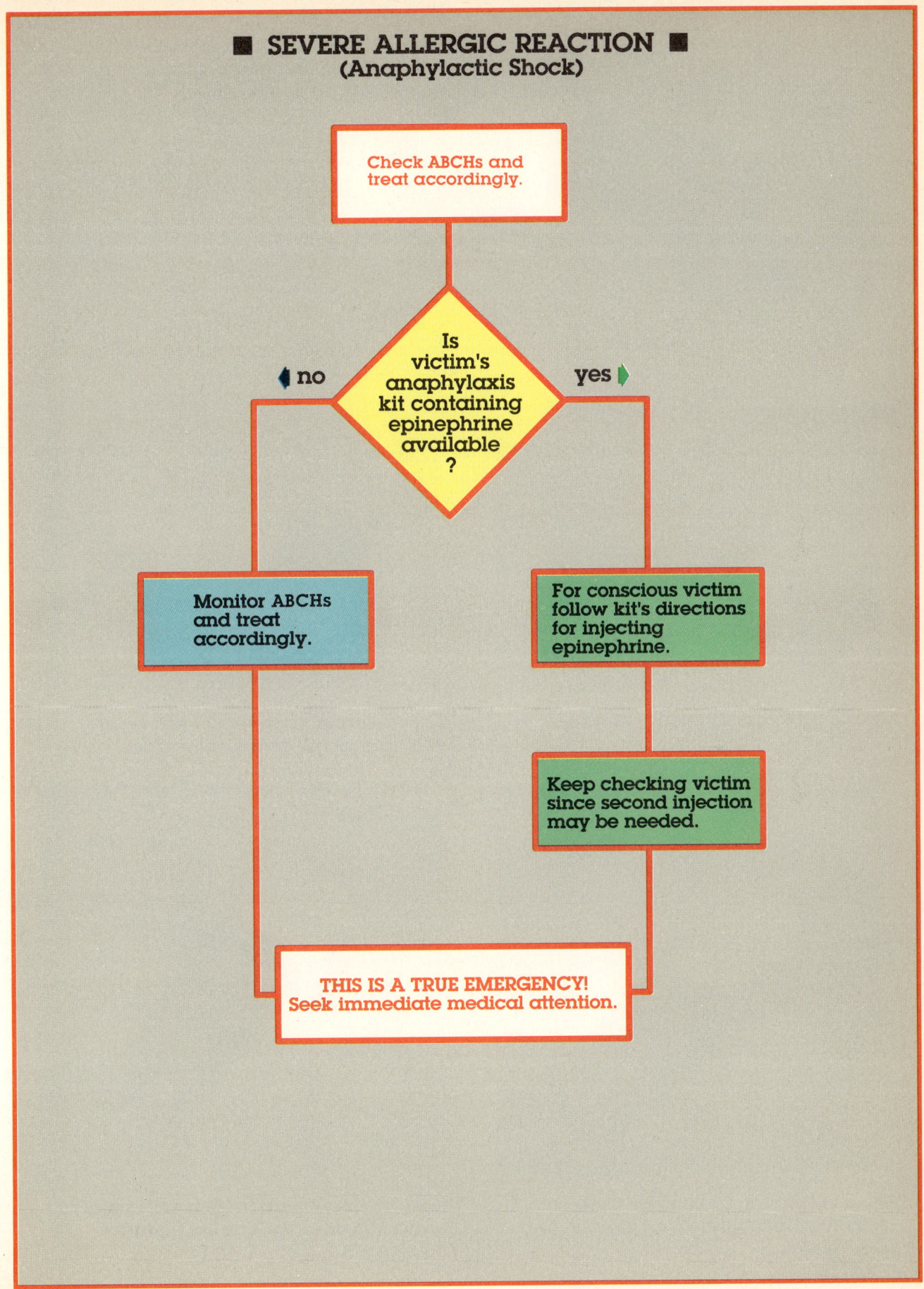

SKILL SCAN: Positioning the Shock Victim

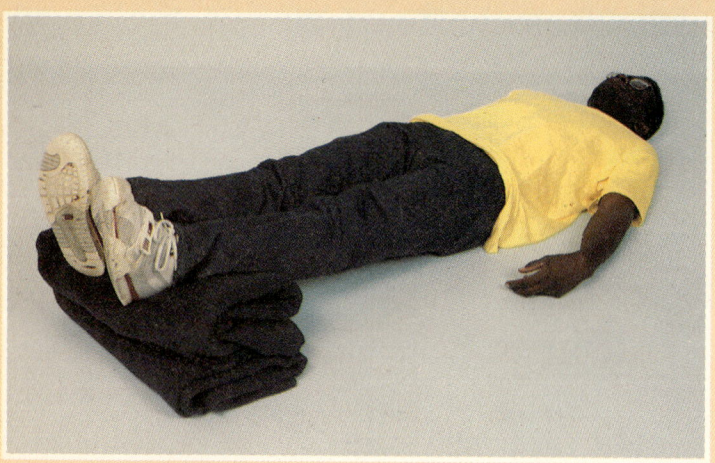

Usual shock position. Elevate the legs 8-12 inches. Do not lift the foot of bed or stretcher.

EXCEPTIONS:

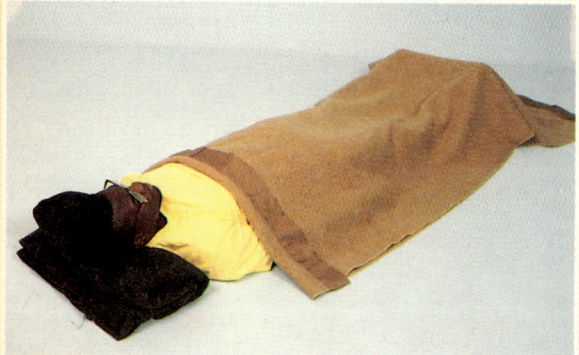

Elevate the head for injuries or stroke.

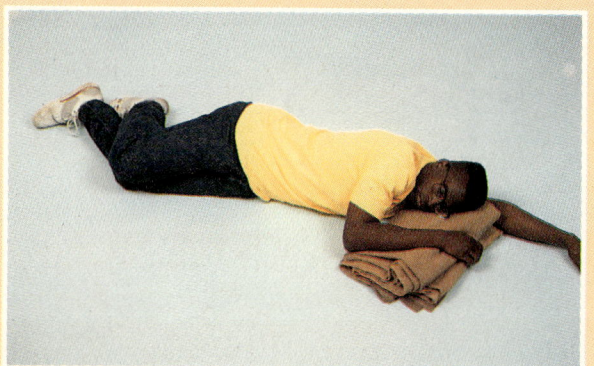

Lay an unconcious, semiconcious, or vomiting victim on his or her side.

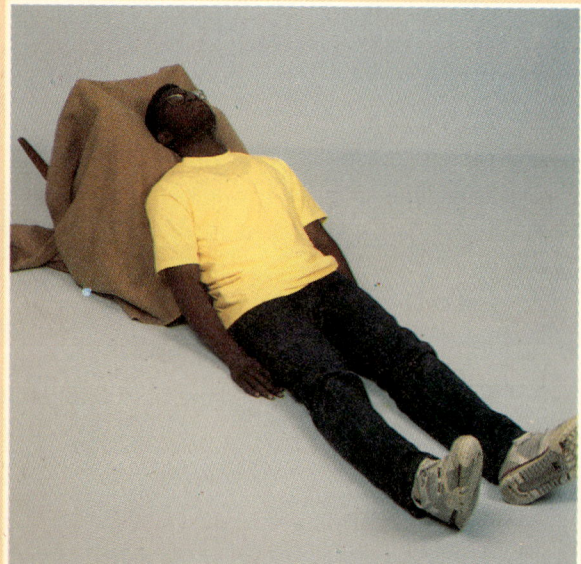

Use a semisitting position for those with breathing difficulties, chest injuries, or a heart attack.

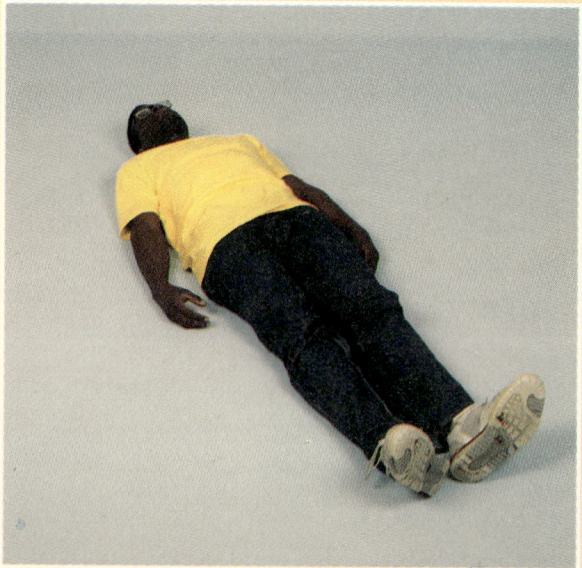

Keep victim flat if a neck or spine injury is suspected or victim has leg fractures.

5
Bleeding and Wounds

The average-sized adult has about six quarts of blood and can safely lose a pint during a blood donation. However, rapid blood loss of one quart or more can lead to shock and death. A child losing one pint is in extreme danger.

Blood can be lost from arteries, veins, or capillaries. Most bleeding involves more than one type of blood vessel. Blood from arteries is bright red and spurts. Arterial bleeding loses blood the fastest, is the most difficult to control, and is therefore the most dangerous.

Blood from a vein flows steadily and appears to be a darker red. Blood oozes slowly from capillaries. Though each blood vessel contains blood differing in shades of red, an inexperienced person may have difficulty detecting the difference. The two basic types of bleeding are external and internal.

External Bleeding

This type involves seeing blood coming from a wound. In most cases, bleeding stops after 5 to 10 minutes with proper first aid.

Internal Bleeding

Bleeding occurs when the skin is unbroken, and is not usually visible.

Signs and Symptoms

- Blood from the mouth (vomit, sputum) or rectum, or blood in the urine
- Nonmenstrual bleeding from the vagina
- Bruise or contusion
- Rapid pulse
- Cold and moist skin
- Dilated pupils
- Nausea and vomiting
- Pain, tender, rigid, bruised abdomen
- Fractured ribs or bruises on chest

Animal and Human Bites

Animal bites rarely cause lethal bleeding, but they can produce significant damage. Sixty to 90% of the animal bites in the United States come from dogs. The annual

TABLE 5-1 Types of Open Wounds

Type	Cause(s)	Signs and Symptoms	First Aid
Abrasion (scrape)	Rubbing or scraping	Only skin surface affected	Remove all debris.
		Little bleeding	Wash away from wound with soap and water.
Incision (cut)	Sharp objects	Smooth edges of wound	Control bleeding.
		Severe bleeding	Wash wound.
Laceration (tearing)	Blunt object tearing skin	Veins and arteries can be affected	Control bleeding.
		Severe bleeding	Wash wound.
		Danger of infection	
Puncture (stab)	Sharp pointed object pierces skin	Wound is narrow and deep into veins and arteries	Do not remove impaled objects.
		Embedded objects	
		Danger of infection	
Avulsion (torn off)	Machinery, Explosives	Tissue torn off or left hanging	Control bleeding.
		Severe bleeding	Take avulsed part to medical facility.

Bloodborne Pathogens: HIV and HBV

Bloodborne pathogens are disease-causing microorganisms that may be present in human blood. They may be transmitted with any exposure to blood. Two significant pathogens are Hepatitis B Virus (HBV) and Human Immunodeficiency Virus (HIV). A number of bloodborne diseases other than HIV and HBV exist, such as Hepatitis C, Hepatitis D, and syphilis. Other body fluids may also spread bloodborne pathogens.

The HBV attacks the liver. HBV is very infectious and can cause:

- Active hepatitis B—a flu-like illness that can last for months
- A chronic carrier state—the person may have no symptoms, but can pass HBV to others
- Cirrhosis, liver cancer, and death

Fortunately, vaccines are available to prevent HBV infection. Even if you are vaccinated against HBV, you must treat all blood and certain human body fluids as if they are known to be infected with bloodborne pathogens (known as the "universal precautions").

HIV causes AIDS (Acquired Immune Deficiency Syndrome). HIV attacks the immune system, making the body less able to fight off infections. In most cases, these infections eventually prove fatal. At present there is no vaccine to prevent infection and no known cure for AIDS.

Use personal protective equipment whenever possible while giving first aid:

1. Keep open wounds covered with dressings to prevent contact with blood.

2. All first aid kits should have several pairs of latex gloves. Use these gloves in every situation involving blood or other body fluids.

3. If latex gloves are not available, use the most waterproof material available or extra gauze dressings to form a barrier.

4. Whenever possible, use a mouth-to-barrier device for protection when doing rescue breathing. Every first aid kit should have one. While saliva is not considered a high risk, there may be blood in the mouth.

A person exposed to blood or other body fluids should:

1. Wash the exposed area immediately with soap and running water. Scrub vigorously with lots of lather.

2. Report the incident promptly, according to your workplace policy.

3. Get medical help, treatment and counseling. If your workplace is covered by OSHA's Bloodborne Standards, ask about getting a confidential medical evaluation, testing, counseling, and treatment.

4. Ask about HBV globulin (HBIG) if you haven't had the HBV vaccine. It can provide short-term protection. It's followed by vaccination againts HBV.

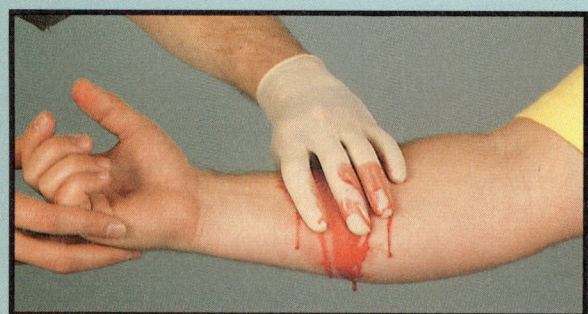

Whenever possible, use gloves as a barrier.

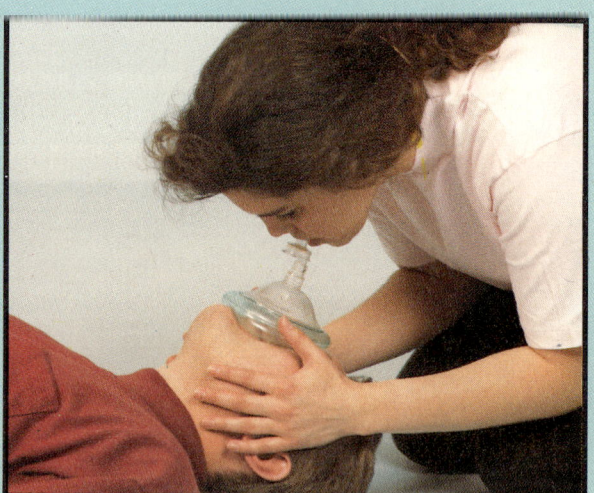

Pocket face mask, one-way valve.

number of dog bites has been estimated to be between one and two million.

Animal bites of all kinds account for about one percent of all hospital emergency department visits. About one bite in 10 needs stitches, but all bites require complete cleaning, which may be impossible for a first aider.

A dog's mouth may carry more than 60 different species of bacteria, some of which are very dangerous to humans (e.g., rabies). Human, cat, and other animal bites are equally contaminated and dangerous.

Human bites can cause very serious injury. The human mouth contains a wide range of bacteria, and the likelihood of infection is greater from a human bite than from other warm-blooded animals.

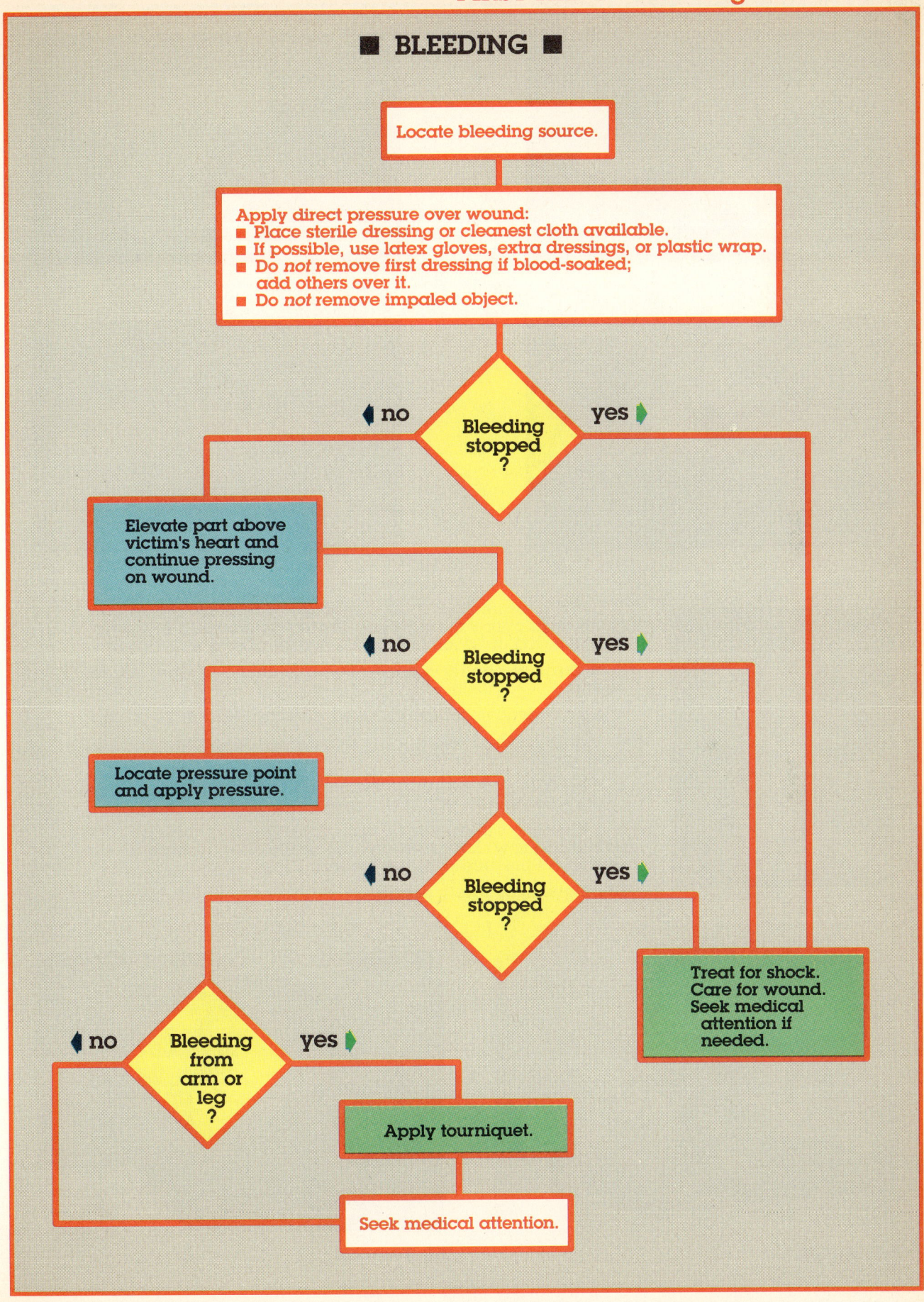

SKILL SCAN: Bleeding Control

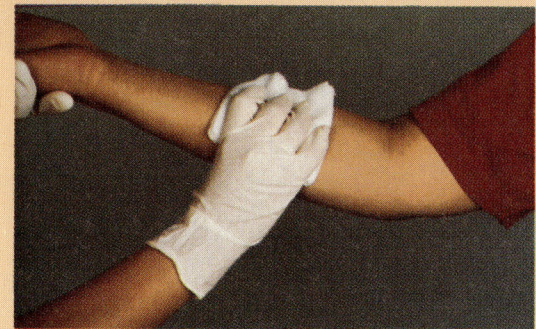

1.

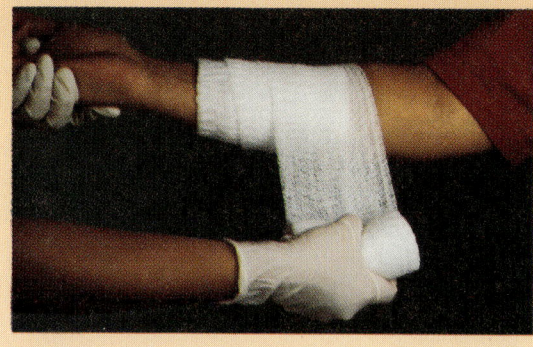

2.

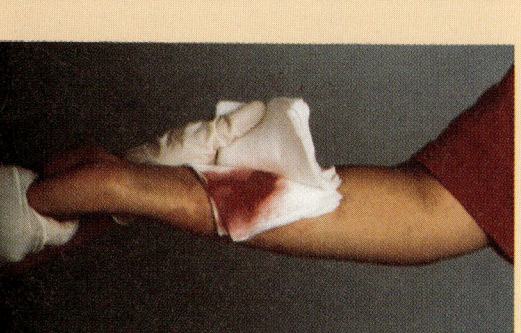

3.

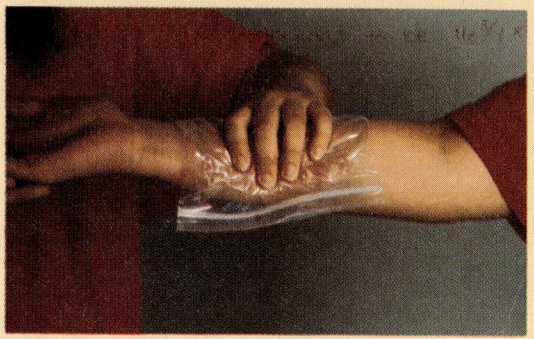

4.

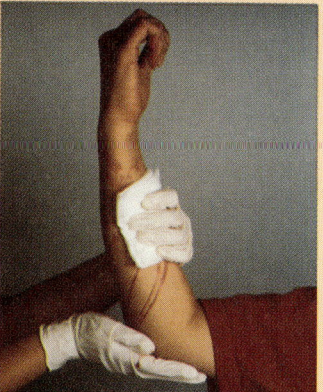

5.

1. Direct pressure stops most bleeding. Place sterile gauze pad or clean cloth over wound. Wear disposable gloves. If bleeding does not stop in 10 minutes, press harder over a wider area.

2. A pressure bandage can free you to attend to other injuries or victims.

3. Do not remove a blood-soaked dressing. Add more on top.

4. If disposable gloves are not available, use another barrier or extra gauze pads or cloths.

5. If bleeding persists, use elevation to help reduce blood flow. It must be combined with direct pressure over the wound.

6. If bleeding still continues, apply pressure at a pressure point to slow blood flow. Locations are: (A) brachial or (B) femoral. Use with direct pressure over the wound.

Tourniquets are rarely needed.

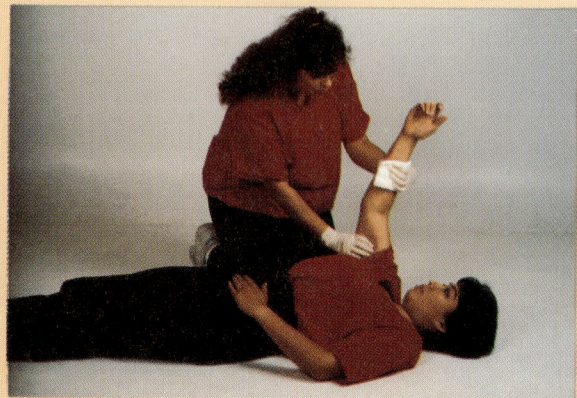

6A. Brachial

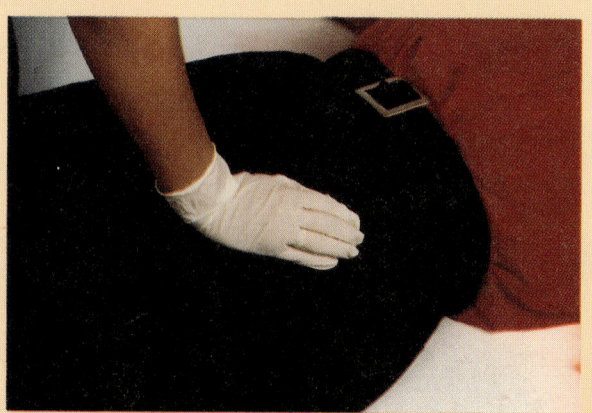

6B. Femoral

6

Specific Body Area Injuries

Head Injuries

Scalp Wounds

Scalp wounds bleed profusely because of the scalp's rich blood supply. Look in the wound for skull bone or brain exposure and indentation of the skull.

Skull Fracture

A skull fracture is a break or crack in the cranium (bony case surrounding the brain). Skull fractures may be open or closed, as with other bone fractures.

Signs and symptoms

- Pain at the point of injury
- Deformity of the skull
- Bleeding from ears and/or nose
- Leakage of clear or pink watery fluid dripping from the nose or ear (This watery fluid is known as cerebrospinal fluid, or CSF. CSF can be detected by having the suspected fluid drip onto a handkerchief, pillowcase, or other cloth. CSF will form a pink ring resembling a target around the blood; this is also called the "halo sign.")
- Discoloration under the eyes ("raccoon eyes.")
- Discoloration behind an ear (Battle's sign)
- Unequal pupils
- Profuse scalp bleeding if skin is broken. A scalp wound may expose skull or brain tissue.

Concussion

A concussion comes from a blow to the head that results in a violent jar or shaking to the brain, causing an immediate change in brain function, including possible loss of consciousness.

Signs and Symptoms

- Loss of consciousness
- Severe headache
- Memory loss (amnesia)
- "Seeing stars"
- Dizziness
- Weakness
- Double vision

TABLE 6-1 Concussion Guidelines

Type	Description	Guidelines
Mild	Momentary or no loss of consciousness	Delay return to activity until medical evaluation has been made.
Moderate	Unconscious for less than five minutes	Avoid vigorous activity for a few days or longer. Resume activity only when associated symptoms of headache, visual disturbances, etc. have been resolved.
Severe	Unconscious for more than five minutes	Avoid rigorous activity for one month or longer. Clearance from a neurosurgeon is advised.

Contusion

Contusions are more serious than concussions. Both can be produced by hits or blows to the head. Contusions involve bruising and swelling of the brain, with blood vessels within the brain rupturing and bleeding. Inside the skull, there is no way for the blood to escape and no room for it to accumulate.

Signs and Symptoms

- Similar to those of a concussion but more severe
- Unconsciousness
- Paralysis or weakness
- Unequal pupil size
- Vomiting and nausea
- Blurred vision
- Amnesia or memory lapses
- Headache

Head Injury Follow-Up

After a head injury, certain signs may indicate a need for medical attention.

- **Headache.** Expect a headache. If it lasts more than one or two days or increases in severity, seek medical advice.
- **Nausea, vomiting.** If nausea lasts more than two hours, seek medical advice. Vomiting once or twice, especially in children, may be expected after a head injury. Vomiting does not tell anything about the severity of the injury. However, if vomiting begins again hours after one or two episodes have ceased, consult a physician.
- **Drowsiness.** Allow a victim to sleep, but wake the victim at least every hour to check the state of consciousness and sense of orientation by asking his or her name, address, telephone number, and whether information can be processed (e.g., adding or multiplying numbers). If the victim cannot answer correctly or appears confused or disoriented, call a physician.
- **Vision problems.** If the victim "sees double," if the eyes fail to move together, or if one pupil appears to be larger than the other, seek medical advice.
- **Mobility.** If victim cannot use his or her arms or legs as well as previously or is unsteady in walking, medical care should be sought.
- **Speech.** If the victim slurs his or her speech or is unable to talk, a doctor should be consulted.
- **Seizures or convulsions.** If the victim's voluntary muscles start to contract involuntarily, seek medical assistance.

Eye Injuries

Correct treatment of an eye injury immediately following an accident can prevent loss of sight. However, because it is difficult to determine the extent of damage to the eye, medical help should be sought as soon as possible. Call an ophthalmologist or a family physician, or go to a nearby hospital emergency department immediately.

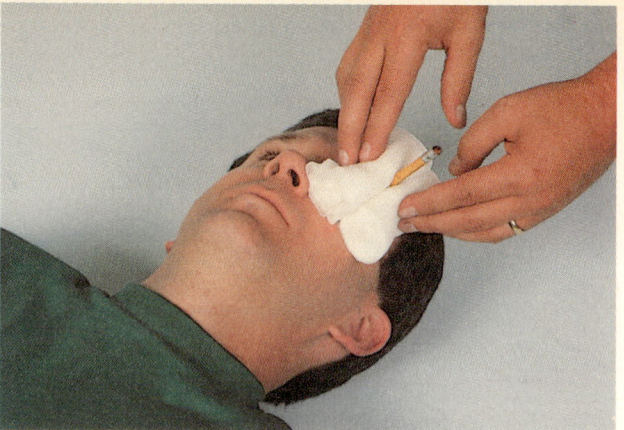
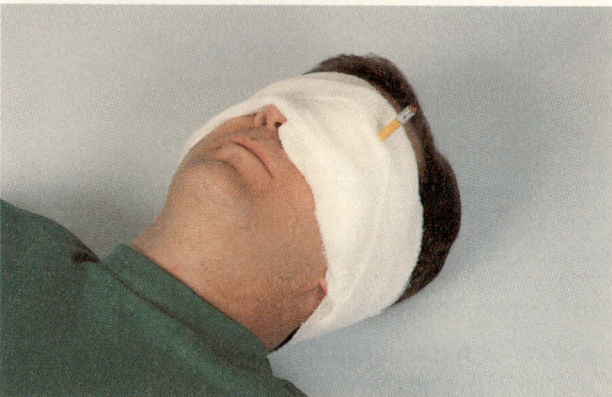
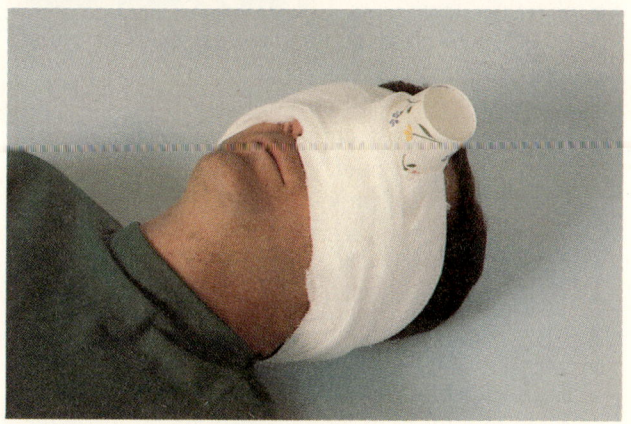

Bandaging eye (paper cup)

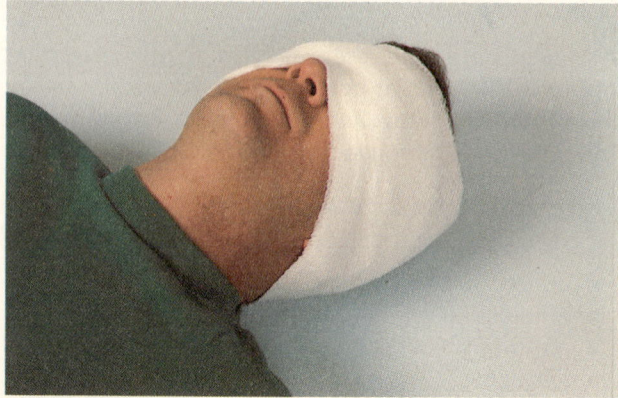

Bandaging both eyes

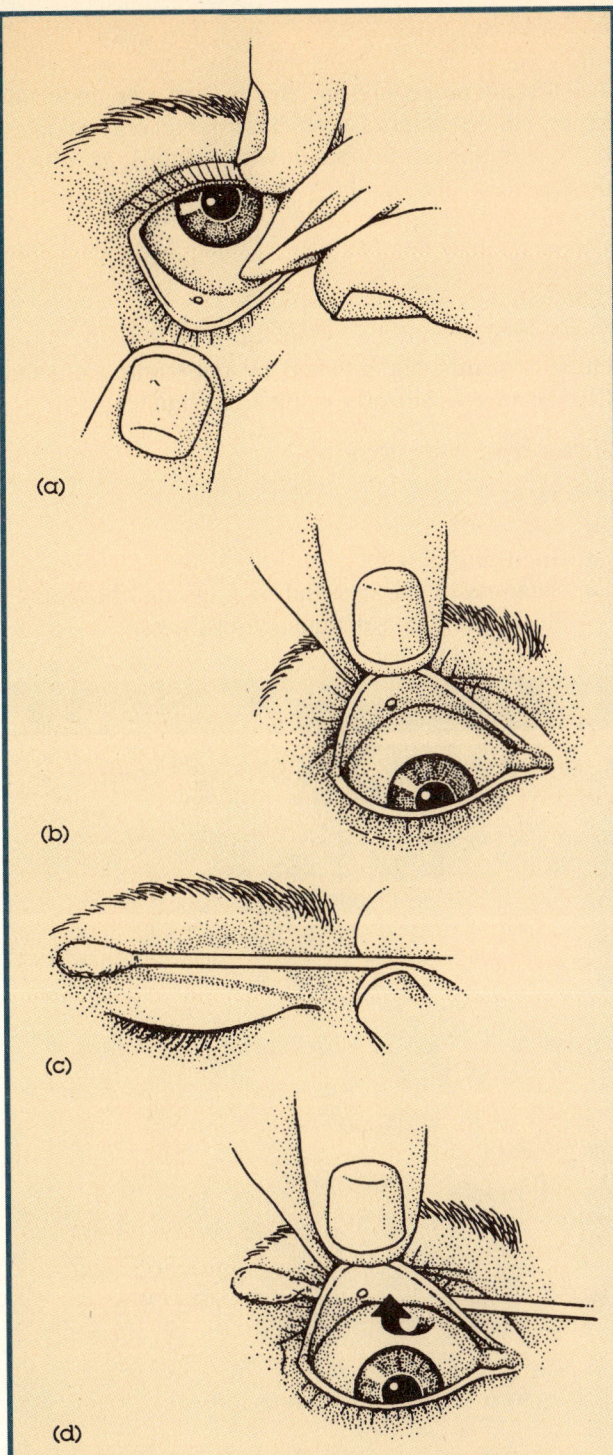

Everted Eyelid a. If tears or gentle flushing do not remove object, gently pull lower lid down. Remove an object by gently flushing with lukewarm water or a wet sterile gauze.
b. If no object is seen inside lower lid, check upper lid. **c.** Tell the person to look down. Pull gently downward on upper eyelashes. Lay a swab or matchstick across the top of the lid.
d. Fold the lid over the swab or matchstick. Remove an object by gently flushing with lukewarm water or a wet sterile gauze.

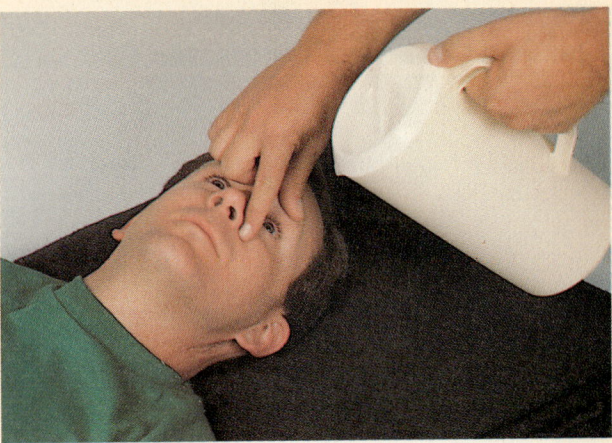

Flushing eye for chemical burn

Nosebleeds

Severe nosebleed frightens the victim and often challenges the first aider's skill. Most nosebleeds are self-limited and seldom require medical attention. However, in cases of accompanying head or neck injuries, stabilize the head and neck for protection. In some cases enough blood could be lost to cause shock.

Types of Nosebleeds

- *Anterior* (front of nose). The most common (90%); bleeds out of one nostril
- *Posterior* (back of nose). Massive bleeding backward into the mouth or down the back of the throat; bleeding starts on one side, then comes out of both sides and down the throat; serious and requires medical attention

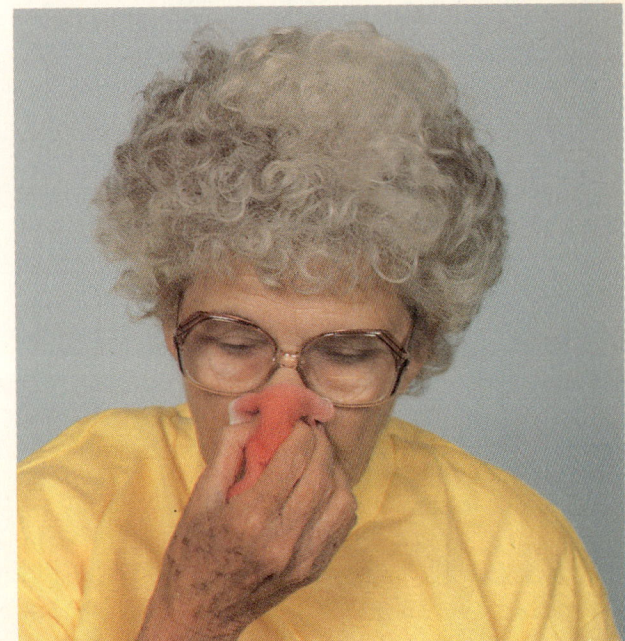

Nosebleed control

Care After a Nosebleed

After a nosebleed has stopped, suggest to the victim:

1. Sneeze through an open mouth if there is a need to sneeze.
2. Do not bend over or exert self physically.
3. Elevate the head with two pillows when lying down.
4. Keep the nostrils moist by applying a little petroleum jelly just inside the nostril for a week and increase the humidity in the bedroom during the winter months with a cold-mist humidifier.
5. Avoid picking or rubbing the nose.
6. Avoid hot drinks and alcoholic beverages for a week.
7. Avoid smoking or taking aspirin for a week.

Dental Injuries

The first aid procedures in Table 6.2 serve as guidelines for providing temporary relief for dental emergencies, but it is important to consult with a dentist as soon as possible.

Chest Injuries

Chest wounds may be either **open** or **closed. Open chest wounds** are inflicted by penetrating objects. **Closed chest wounds** result from blunt blows.

Signs and Symptoms

Important signs of chest injuries include:
- Pain at the injury site
- Breathing difficulty
- Blueness of the lips and/or fingernail beds, indicating oxygen deficiency (cyanosis)

TABLE 6-2 Dental Emergency Procedures

Toothache	Rinse the mouth vigorously with warm water to clean it out. Use dental floss to remove any food that might be trapped between the teeth. (*Do not place aspirin on the aching tooth or gum tissues.*) See the dentist as soon as possible.
Problems with braces and retainers	If a wire is causing irritation, cover the end with a small cotton ball, beeswax or a piece of gauze, until you can get to the dentist.
	If a wire gets stuck in the cheek, tongue or gum tissue, do not attempt to remove it. Go to the dentist immediately.
	If an appliance becomes loose or a piece of it breaks off, take the appliance and the piece and go to the dentist.
Knocked-out tooth	If the tooth is dirty, rinse it gently in running water. *Do not scrub it or remove any attached tissue fragments.*
	Gently insert and hold the tooth in its socket. If this is not possible, place the tooth in a cup of milk or a special tooth-preserving solution available at your local drugstore.
	If you can get to the dentist within 30 minutes, there is a good chance the tooth can be saved! Do not forget to bring the tooth!
Broken tooth	Gently clean dirt from the injured area with warm water. Place cold compresses on the face, in the area of the injured tooth, to decrease swelling.
	Go to the dentist immediately.
Bitten tongue or lip	Apply direct pressure to the bleeding area with a clean cloth. If swelling is present, apply cold compresses. If bleeding does not stop, go to a hospital emergency room.
Objects wedged between teeth	Try to remove the object with floss. Guide the floss carefully to avoid cutting the gums. If you're not successful in removing the object, go to the dentist. Do not try to remove the object with a sharp or pointed instrument.
Possible broken jaw	Do not move the jaw. Secure the jaw in place by tying a handkerchief, necktie or towel around the jaw and over the top of the head. If swelling is present, apply cold compresses. Go immediately to a hospital or emergency room, or call your dentist.

Source: Copyright by the American Dental Association; reprinted by permission.

- Coughing or spitting up blood
- Bruising or an open chest wound
- Failure of one or both sides of the chest to expand normally when inhaling

Abdominal Injuries

Abdominal injuries may be **open** or **closed**. **Open injuries** occur when a foreign object enters the abdomen, resulting in external bleeding. **Closed injuries** result from a severe blow that shows no open wound or bleeding on the outside of the body.

Hollow organ (e.g., stomach, intestines) ruptures spill their contents into the abdominal cavity, causing inflammation. Solid organ (e.g., liver, pancreas) ruptures result in severe bleeding.

Signs and Symptoms

- Pain in the abdomen, which may involve cramping
- Legs drawn up to the chest
- Skin wounds and penetrations
- Nausea and vomiting
- Protruding organs
- Blood in the urine or stool
- Guarding abdomen
- Rapid pulse
- Moist, cold skin

Blisters

A blister results from excessive rubbing and is a collection of fluid in a "bubble" under the outer layer of skin. If not infected, blisters usually heal in three to seven days. (This section does *not* cover blisters from burns, frostbite, or contact with a poisonous plant.)

Signs and Symptoms

- Fluid collection under the skin's outer layer
- Pain resulting from touch or pressure
- Swelling and redness around the blister

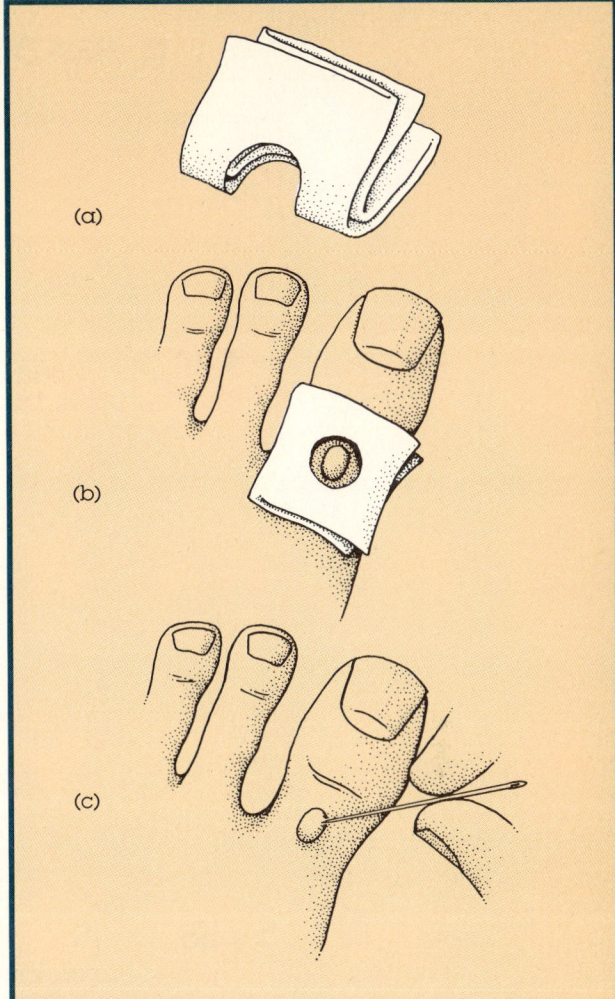

Blister Care a. For unbroken blister, cut holes in several gauze pads. **b.** Stack the pads on the skin with the holes over the blister. Loosely tape an uncut gauze pad over the top. **c.** If blister is painful or likely to break, puncture the blister's edge with a sterilized needle. Drain all the fluid. Tape a sterile or clean gauze pad or cloth over the flattened blister.

FIRST AID 6: Specific Body Area Injuries

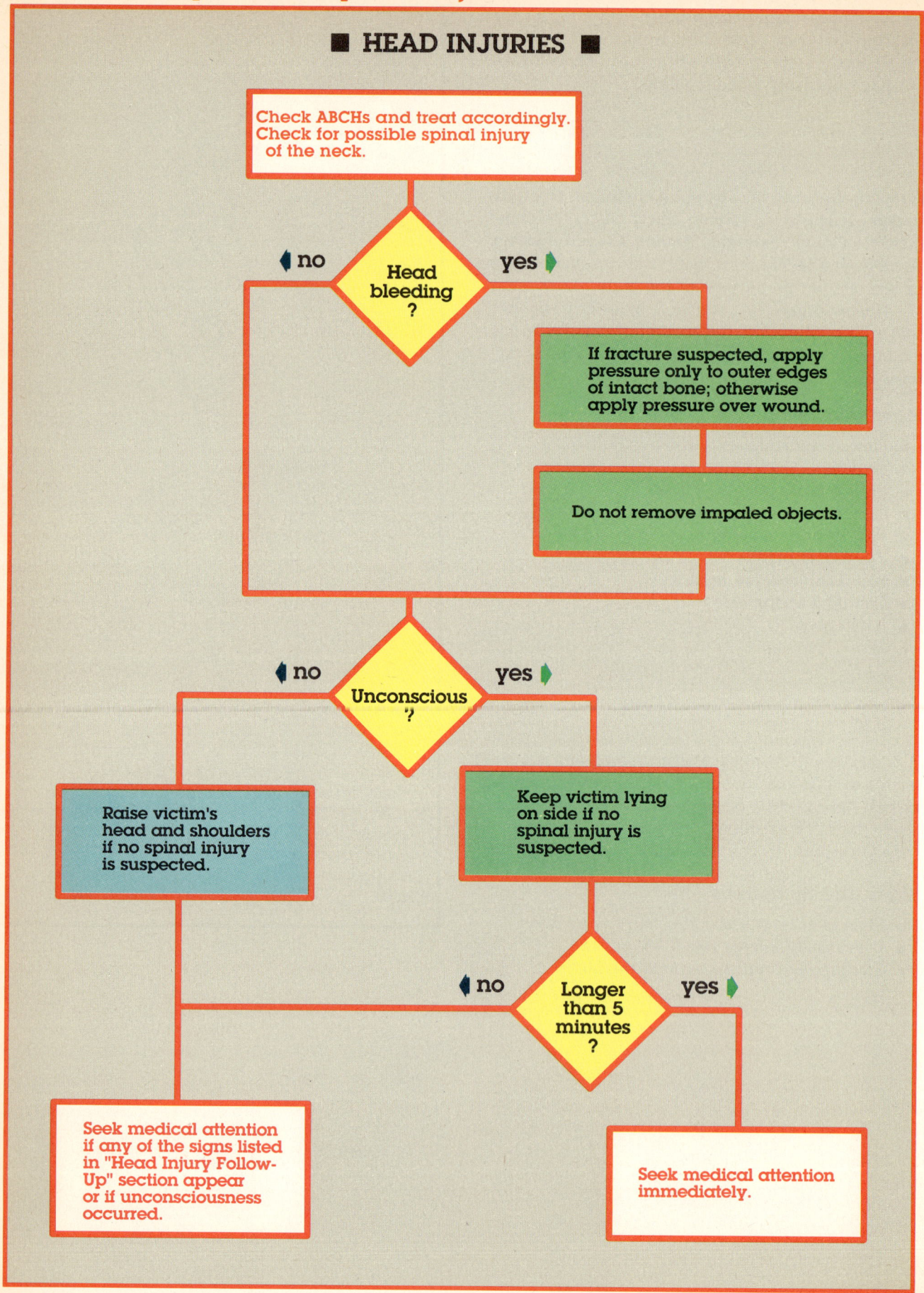

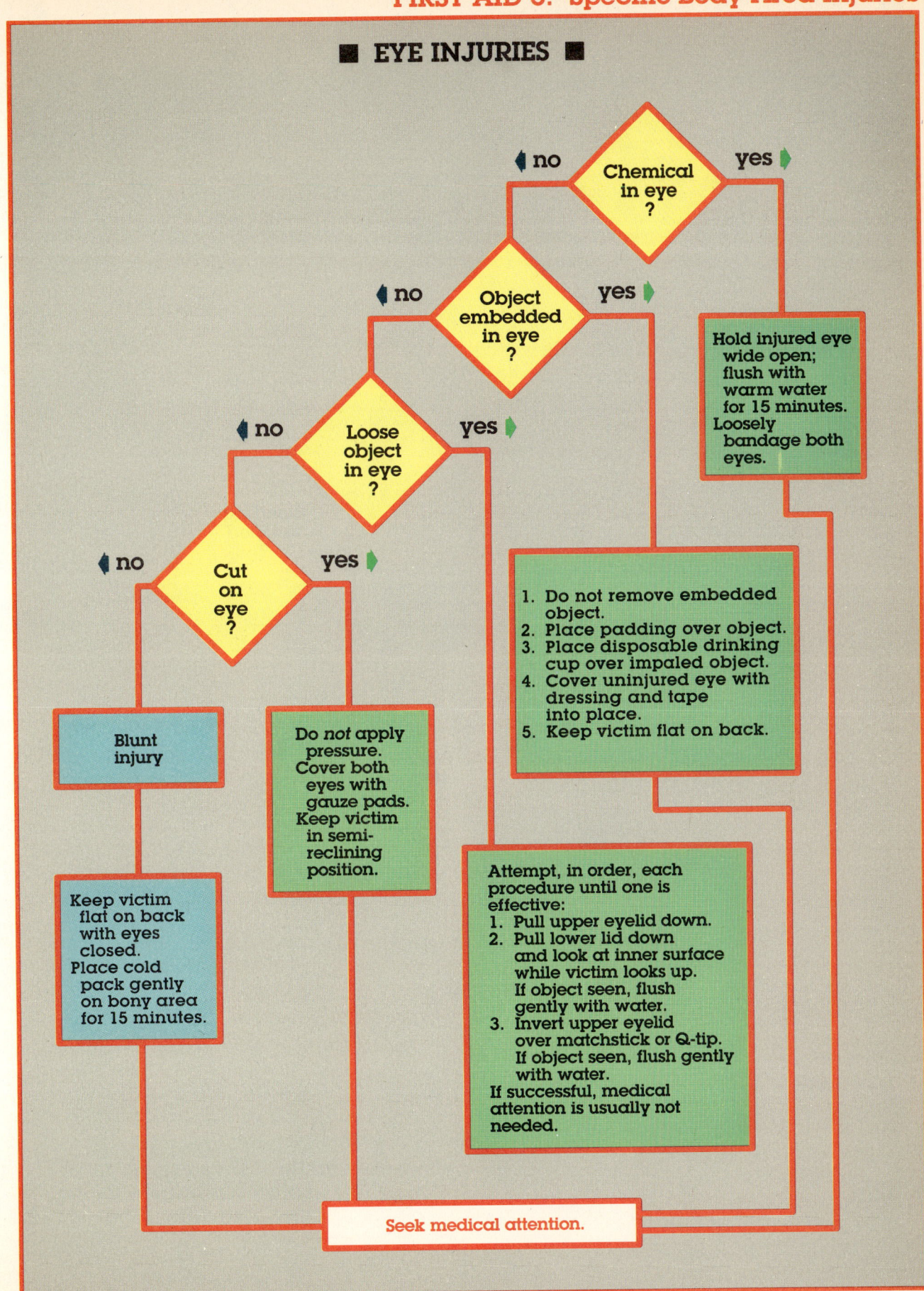

FIRST AID 6: Specific Body Area Injuries

■ NOSEBLEEDS ■

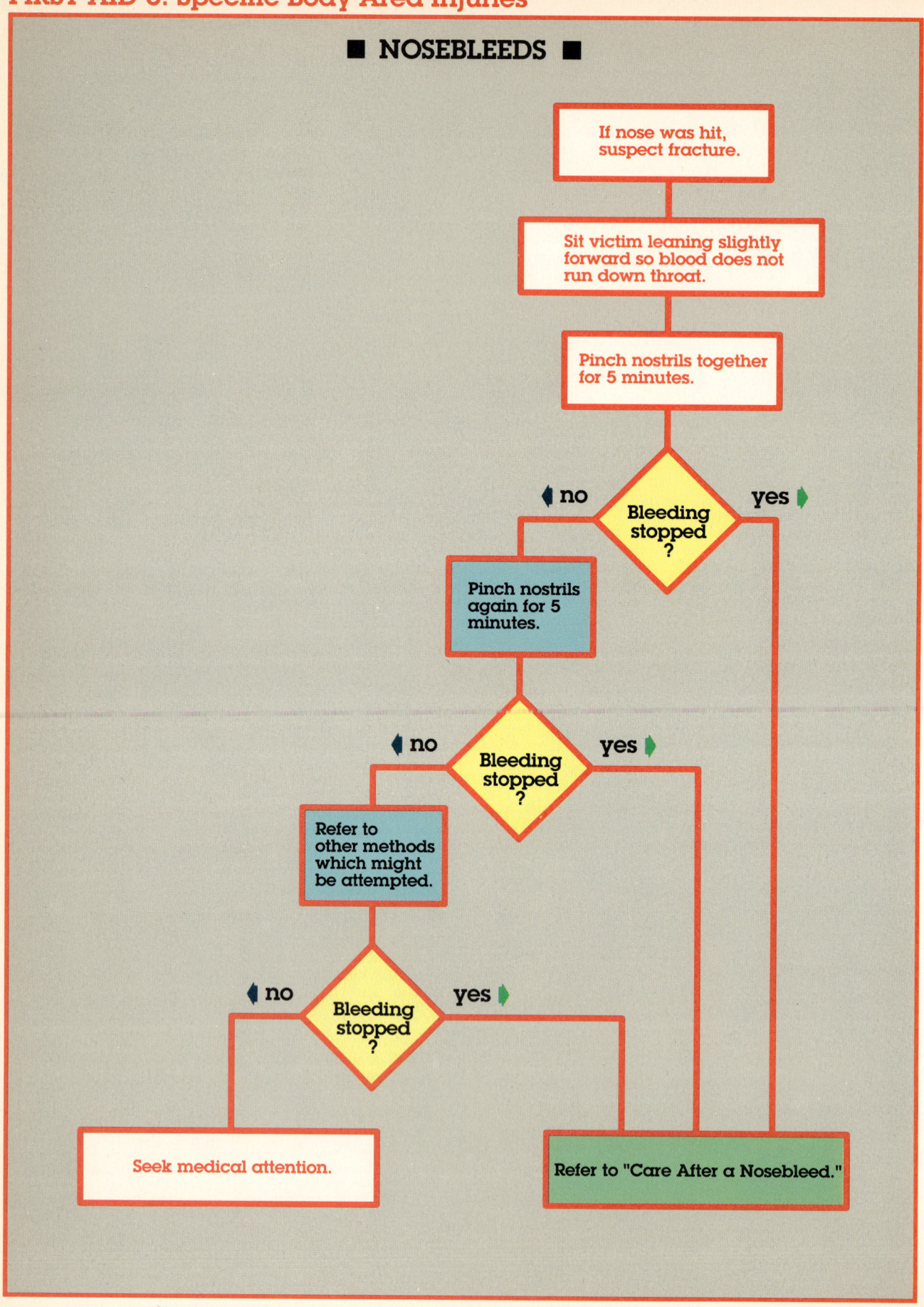

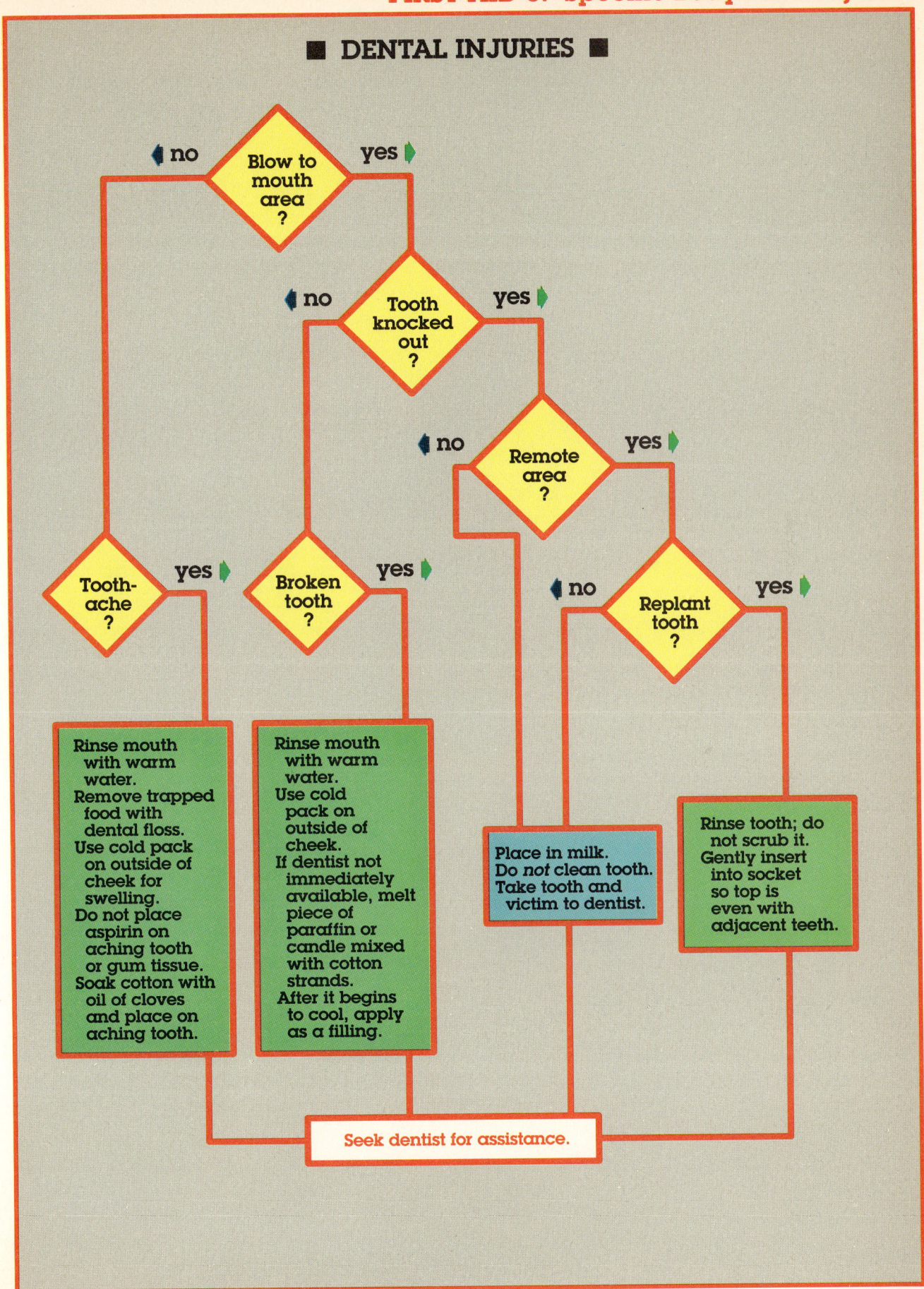

FIRST AID 6: Specific Body Area Injuries

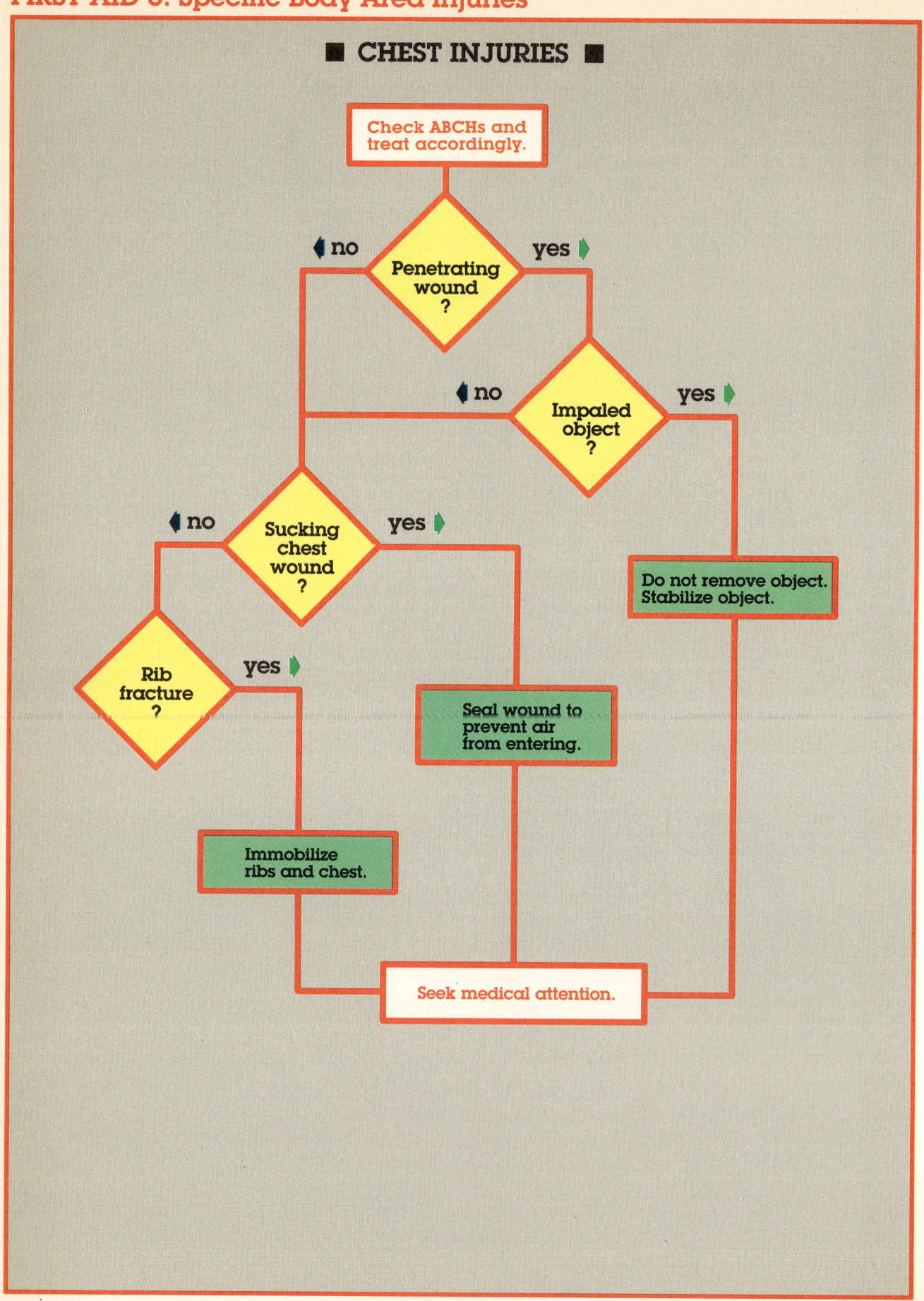

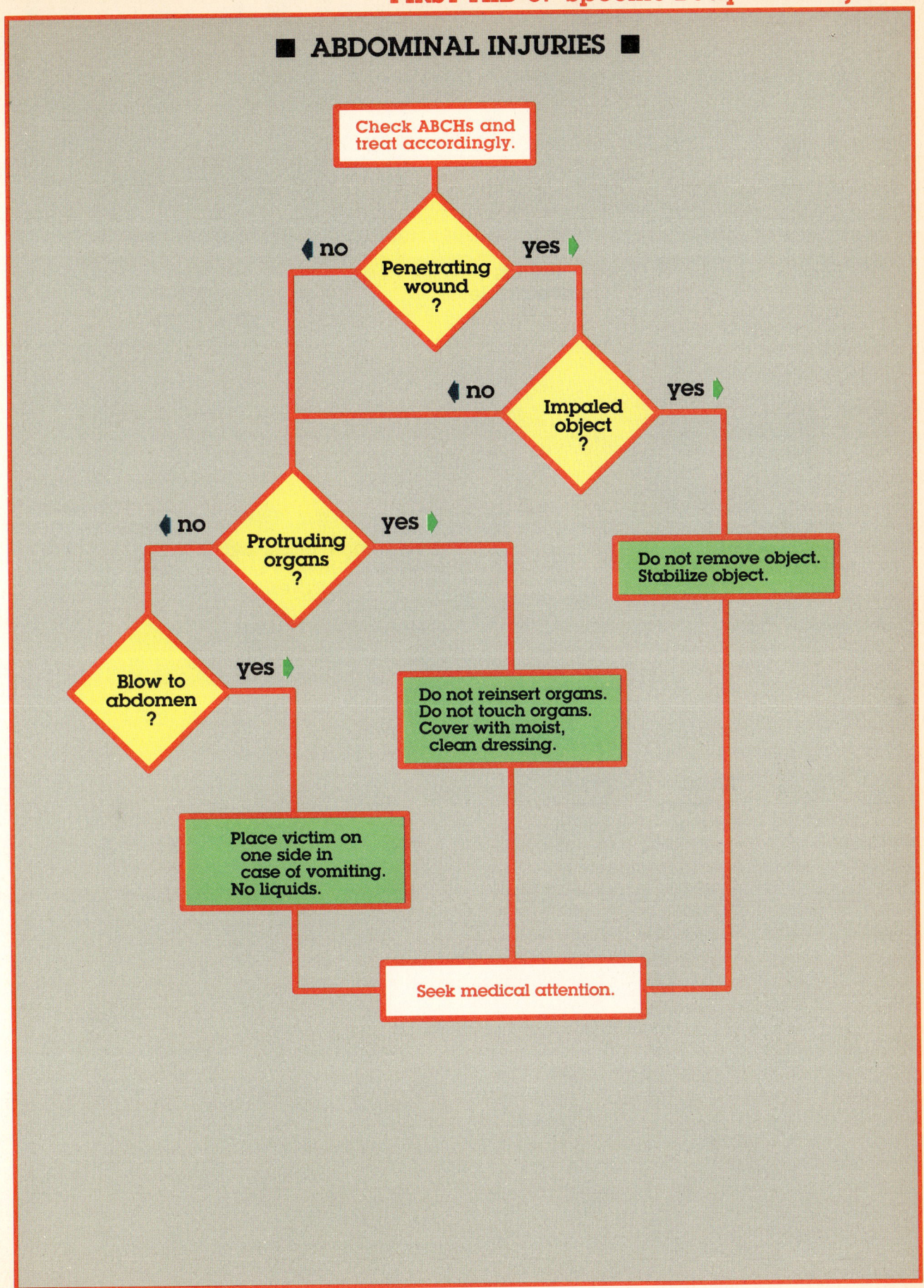

FIRST AID 6: Specific Body Area Injuries

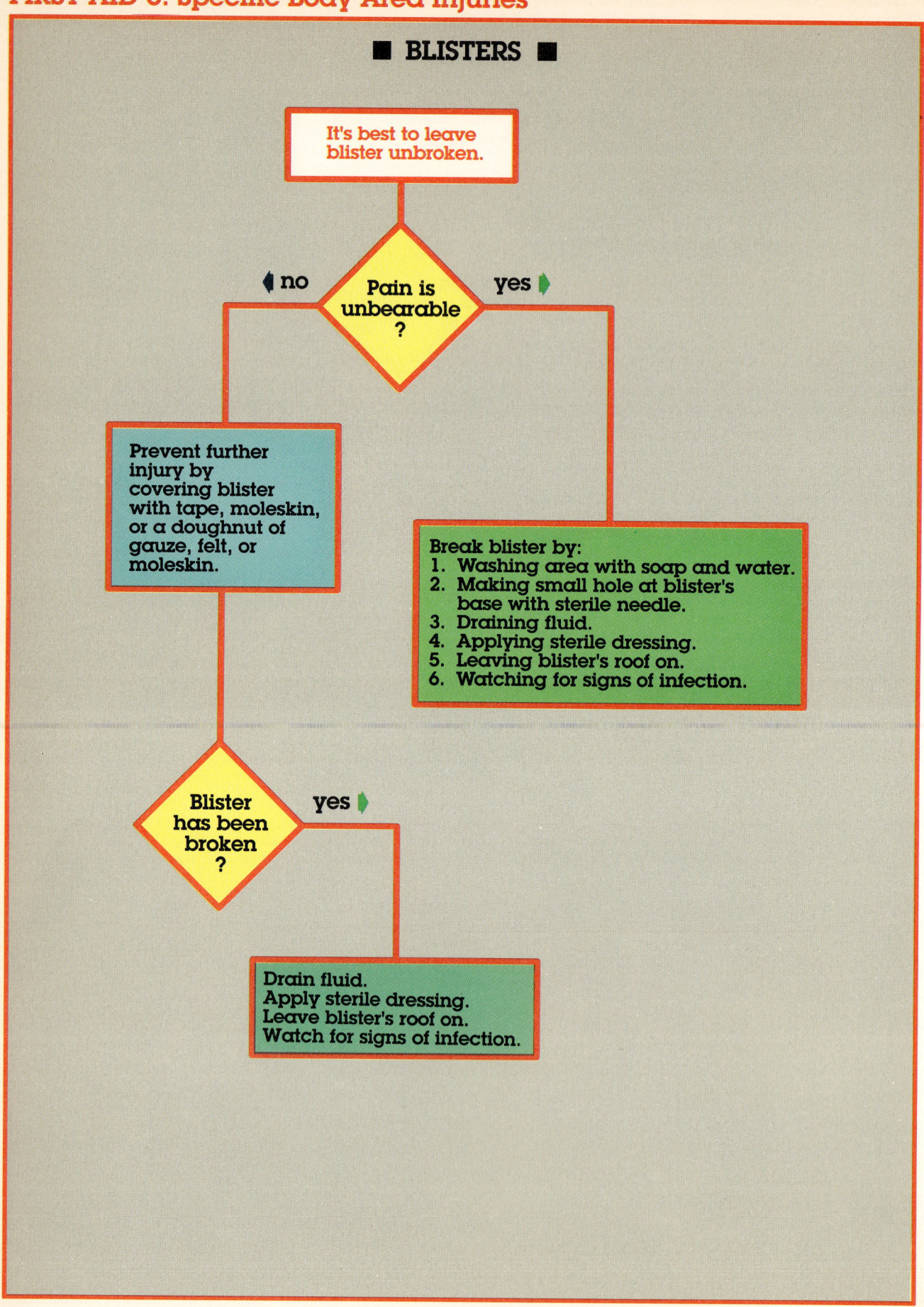

7

Poisoning

Swallowed Poison

A poison is a relatively small amount of any substance (solid, liquid, or gas) that when swallowed, inhaled, absorbed, or injected can by its chemical action damage tissue or adversely change organ function and thus can affect health or cause death.

Deaths by swallowing poisoning have dramatically decreased in recent years, particularly in children under the age of five. Despite this reduction, nonfatal poisoning remains a major cause of hospital admissions and emergency room care. For every poisoning death among children under the age of five, 80,000 to 90,000 nonfatal cases are seen in emergency rooms and about 20,000 children are hospitalized.

Signs and Symptoms

- Abdominal pain and cramping
- Nausea or vomiting
- Diarrhea
- Burns, odor, stains around and in mouth
- Drowsiness or unconsciousness
- Poison containers or plants nearby

Determine the critical information, which includes:

1. *Who?* Age and size of the victim
2. *What?* Type of poison swallowed
3. *How much?* A taste, half a bottle, etc.
4. *How?* Circumstances
5. *When?* Time taken

Contact the poison control center, hospital emergency department, or a physician immediately. Some poisons produce little damage until hours later, while others do damage immediately. More than 70% of poisonings can be treated through instructions taken over the telephone. Otherwise, victims should be transported to a medical facility.

Insect Stings

For a severely allergic person, a single sting may be fatal within 15 minutes. Although accounts exist of individuals who have survived some 2,000 stings, generally 500 or more stings will kill people who are not allergic to stinging insects.

Some experts report that 1% of all children and 4% of adults have such an allergy. An estimated 50–100 sting-related deaths occur yearly. The number of cases may actually be higher but not reported as involving insect stings because they are mistaken for hearts attacks or naturally caused death.

Signs and Symptoms

- *Usual reactions.* Momentary pain, redness around sting site, itching, heat
- *Worrisome reactions.* Skin flush, hives, localized swelling of lips or tongue, "tickle" in throat, wheezing, abdominal cramps, diarrhea
- *Life-threatening reactions.* Bluish or grayish skin color (cyanosis), seizures, unconsciousness, inability to breathe due to swelling of vocal cords

Those who have had a reaction to an insect sting should be instructed in self-treatment so they can protect themselves from severe reactions. They should also be advised to purchase a medical alert bracelet or necklace identifying them as insect-allergic.

Snakebites

Throughout the world about 50,000 people die each year from snakebite. In the United States, of the 40,000 to 50,000 annually bitten, over 7,000 are bitten by poisonous snakes. Amazingly, only a dozen Americans die each year.

Of the many different snake species, only four in the United States are poisonous: rattlesnake, copperhead, water moccasin, and coral snake. The first three are known as pit vipers. They have three common characteristics:

- Triangular, flat head wider than its neck
- Elliptical pupils (e.g., cat's eye)
- Heat-sensitive "pit" located between each eye and nostril

The coral snake is small and very colorful, with a series of bright red, yellow, and black bands around its body. Every other band is yellow. A black snout also marks the coral snake.

Pit Vipers

(rattlesnake, copperhead, water moccasin)

Signs and Symptoms

- Severe burning pain at the bite site
- Two small puncture wounds about 1/2 inch apart (some cases may have only one puncture wound)
- Swelling (happens within 5 minutes and can involve an entire extremity)
- Discoloration and blood-filled blisters
- In severe cases: nausea, vomiting, sweating, weakness
- No venom injected into the victim in about 25% of all poisonous snakebite cases, only fang and tooth wounds

Most snakebites occur within a few hours of a medical facility where antivenin is available. Bites showing no sign of venom injection require only a possible tetanus shot and care of the bite wounds (in the absence of pain or swelling).

Controversy exists about proper first aid procedures for snakebite.

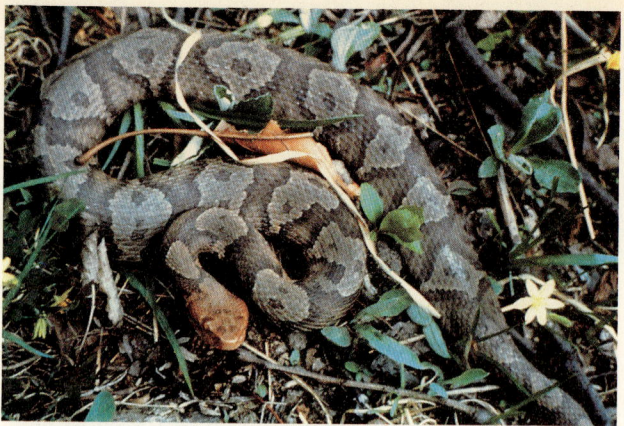
Copperhead snake

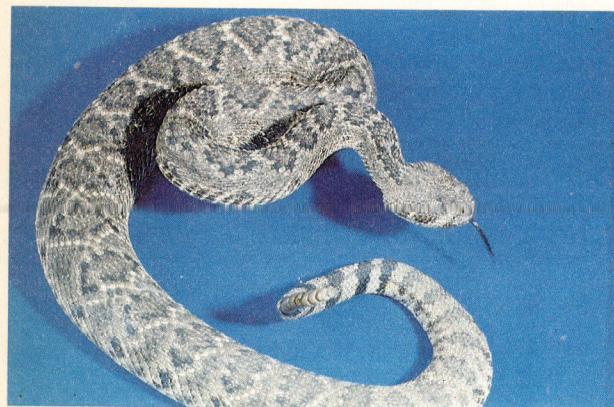
Rattlesnake

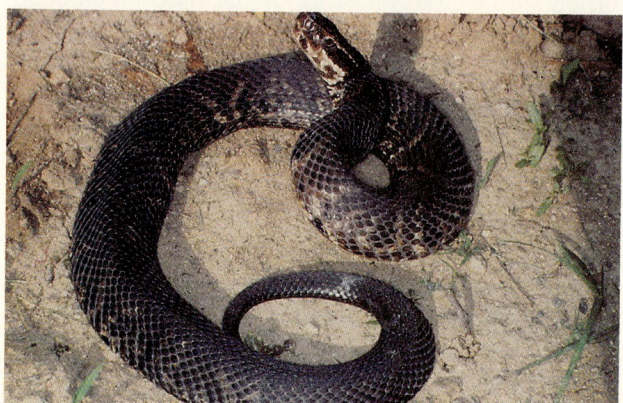
Cottonmouth water moccasin

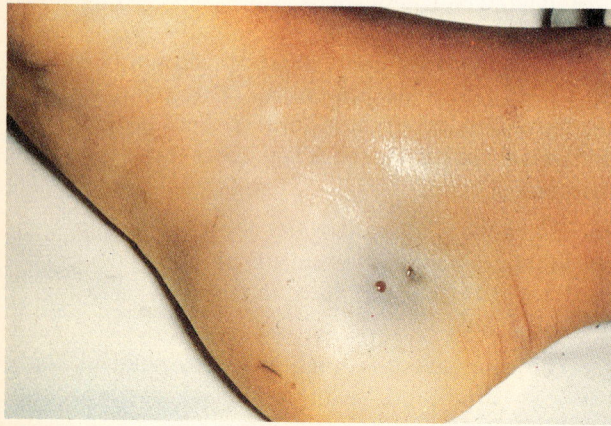
Rattlesnake bite. Note two fang marks.

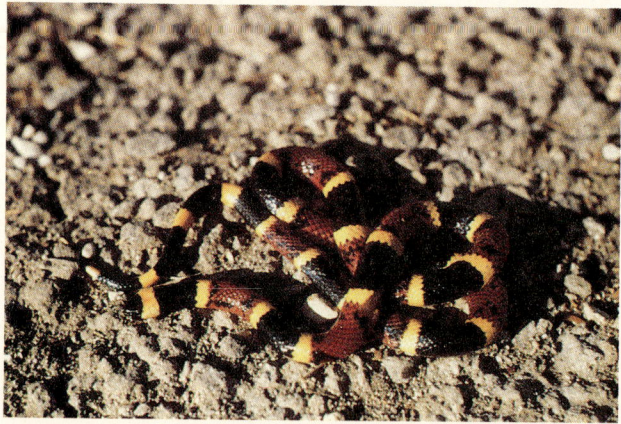
Coral snake, America's most poisonous snake

Spider Bites

Two spiders, the black widow and the brown recluse, can be deadly.

Black Widow Spider

The black widow spider is found throughout the world. A red spot (often in the shape of an hourglass) on the abdomen identifies the female—she is the one that

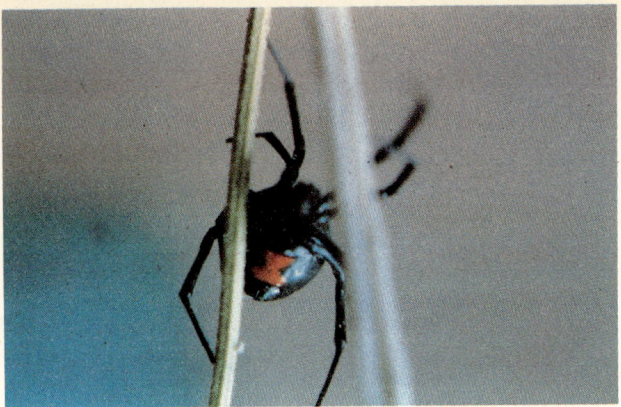

Black widow spider. Note red hour-glass configuration on abdomen.

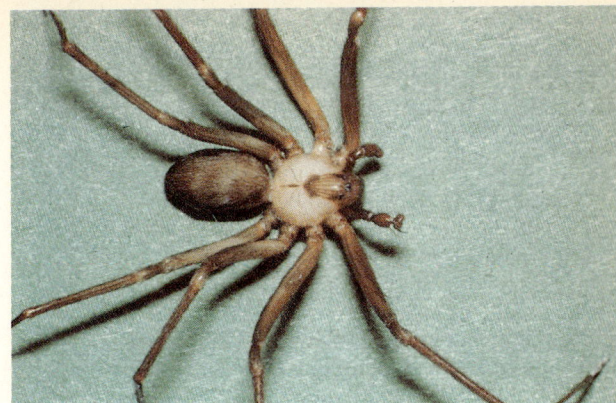

Brown recluse spider. Note violin or fiddle configuration on back.

bites. Females have a glossy black body. By volume, black widow spider venom is more deadly than the rattlesnake's, but it is injected in much smaller amounts.

Signs and Symptoms

Determining whether a person has been bitten by a black widow spider is difficult.

- A sharp pinprick of the spider's bite may be felt, although some victims are not even aware of the bite. In no more than 15 minutes, a dull, numbing pain develops in the bitten extremity.
- Faint red bite marks appear.
- Muscle stiffness and cramps occur next, usually affecting the abdomen when the bite is in the lower part of the body or legs, and affecting the shoulders, back, or chest when the bite is on the upper body or arms.
- Headache, chills, fever, heavy sweating, dizziness, nausea, vomiting, and severe abdominal pain afflict the victim.

Brown Recluse Spider

The brown recluse spider has a brown, possibly purplish, violin-shaped figure on its back. Brown recluse bites are rarely fatal, except for hypersensitive people or for children, the elderly, and those with chronic health problems.

Signs and Symptoms

- The initial pain felt may be slight enough to be overlooked.
- A blister at the bite site, along with redness and swelling, appears after several hours.
- Pain, which may remain mild but can become severe, develops within two to eight hours at the bite site.
- Fever, weakness, vomiting, joint pain, and a rash may occur.

- An ulcer forms within a week. Gangrene may develop in some cases.

Tarantula Spider

More menacing-looking than black widow and brown recluse spiders, the tarantula has a bite that rarely produces symptoms other than mild to moderate pain.

Scorpion Stings

Death from scorpion stings in the United States is rare; children are at greatest risk. A scorpion's sting causes immediate pain and burning around the sting site, followed by numbness or tingling. Severe cases may include paralysis, spasms, or respiratory difficulties.

Tick Bites

Most tick bites are harmless, though ticks can carry serious diseases (e.g., Lyme disease, Rocky Mountain spotted fever, Colorado tick fever). Ticks should be removed as soon as possible.

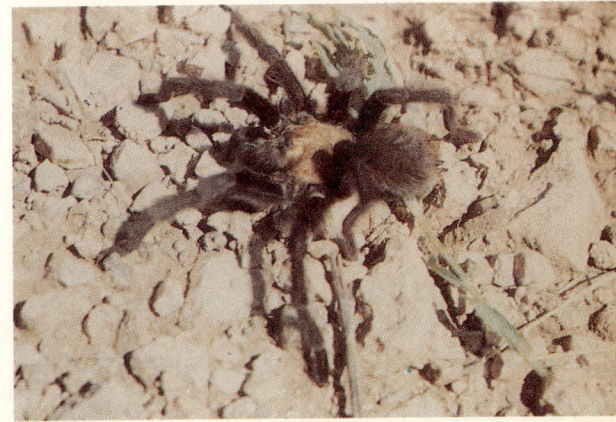

Tarantula

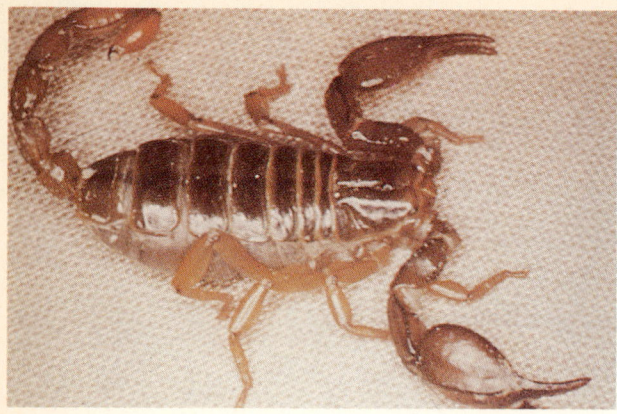
Scorpion

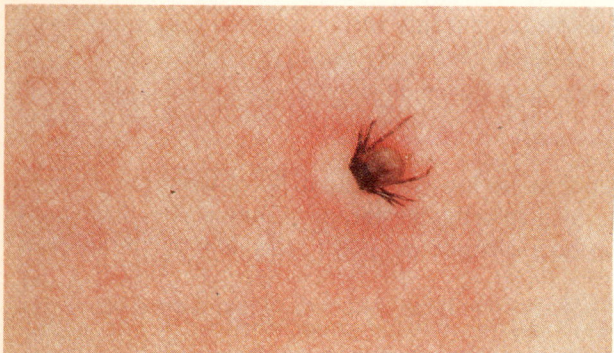
Tick embedded

Poison Ivy, Oak, and Sumac

Poison ivy, oak, and sumac plants cause contact dermatitis or an allergic reaction in about 90% of all adults. Most people cannot recognize these plants. To test a plant for poison, use the "black spot test." Perform this test by crushing the suspected plant's leaf. The sap of poison ivy or oak turns dark brown in 10 minutes and black in one day. Actually, more than 60 plants can cause an allergic reaction, but the three named above are by far the most common offenders.

Allergic people may come in contact with the juice of these plants from their clothes or shoes, from pet fur, or from smoke of burning plants. No one can develop the dermatitis by touching the fluid from blisters, since that fluid does not contain the oleoresin that comes from the juice of these poisonous plants.

Signs and Symptoms

- *Mild.* Some itching
- *Mild to moderate.* Itching and redness
- *Moderate.* Itching, redness, and swelling
- *Severe.* Itching, redness, swelling, and blisters

Severity is important but so is the amount of skin affected. The greater the skin involvement, the greater the need for medical attention. A day or two is the usual time between contact and the onset of the above signs and symptoms.

Carbon Monoxide

Victims of carbon monoxide (CO) are often unaware of its presence. The gas is invisible, tasteless, odorless, and nonirritating.

Carbon monoxide produces its toxicity due to several factors. CO becomes tightly bound to hemoglobin (red blood cells) that carries oxygen. With conscious victims it takes four to five hours with ordinary air (21% oxygen) or 30–40 minutes with 100% oxygen to reverse CO's effects. When CO levels in the air are high, the level of oxygen is probably low.

Signs and Symptoms

It is difficult to tell if a person is a victim of carbon monoxide poisoning. Sometimes, a complaint of having the flu is really a symptom of carbon monoxide poisoning.
- Headache
- Ringing in the ears (tinnitus)
- Angina (chest pain)
- Muscle weakness
- Nausea and vomiting
- Dizziness and visual changes (blurred or double vision)
- Unconsciousness
- Breathing and cardiac failure

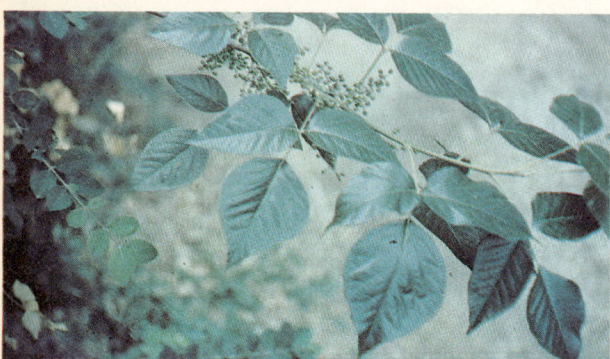
Poison ivy, found in all 48 contiguous U.S. states

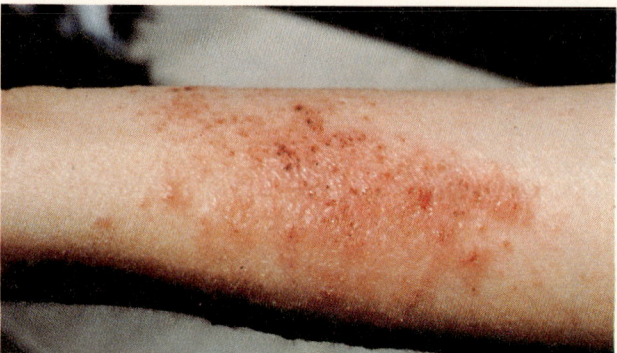
Poison ivy dermatitis

FIRST AID 7: Poisoning

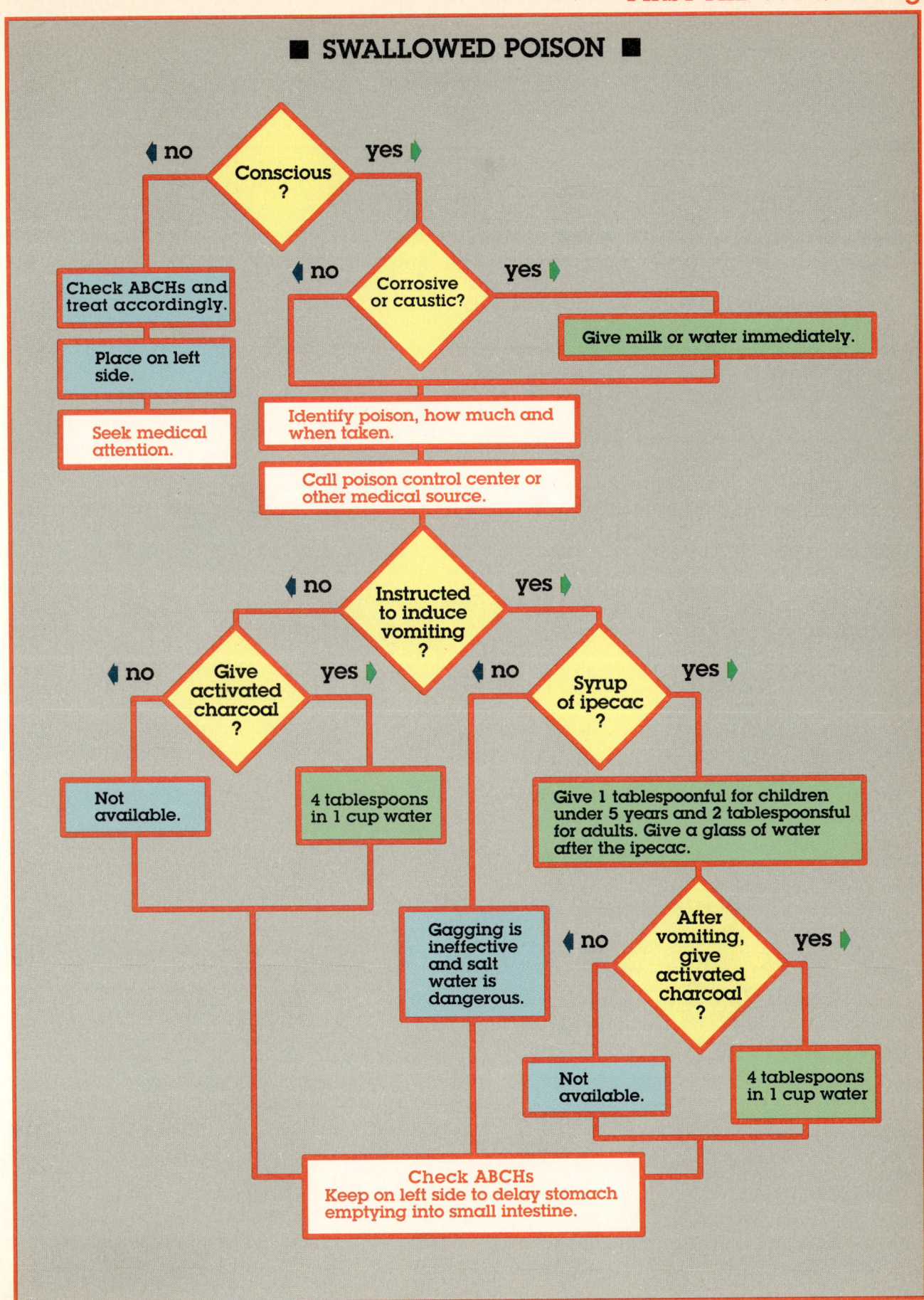

FIRST AID 7: Poisoning

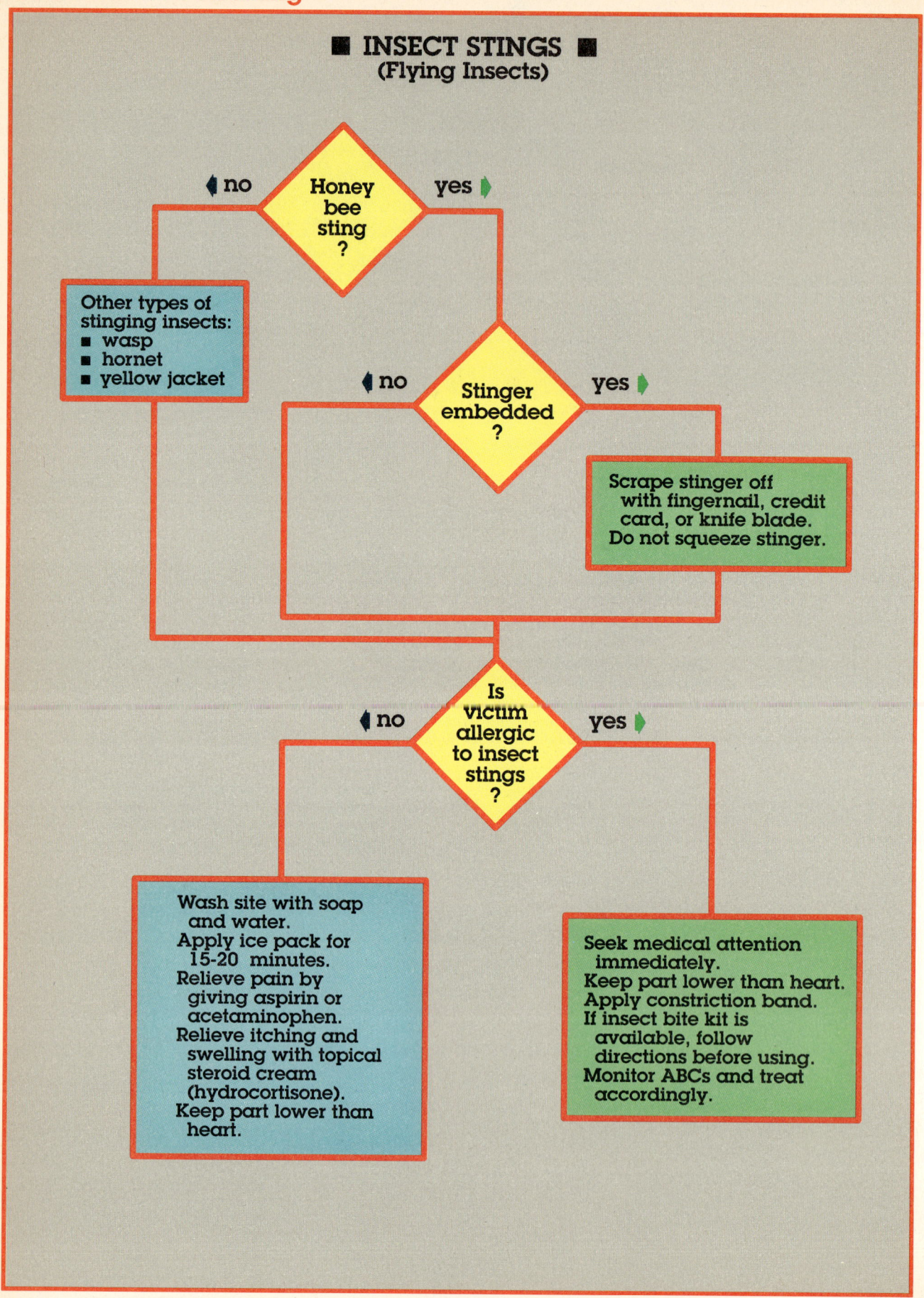

FIRST AID 7: Poisoning

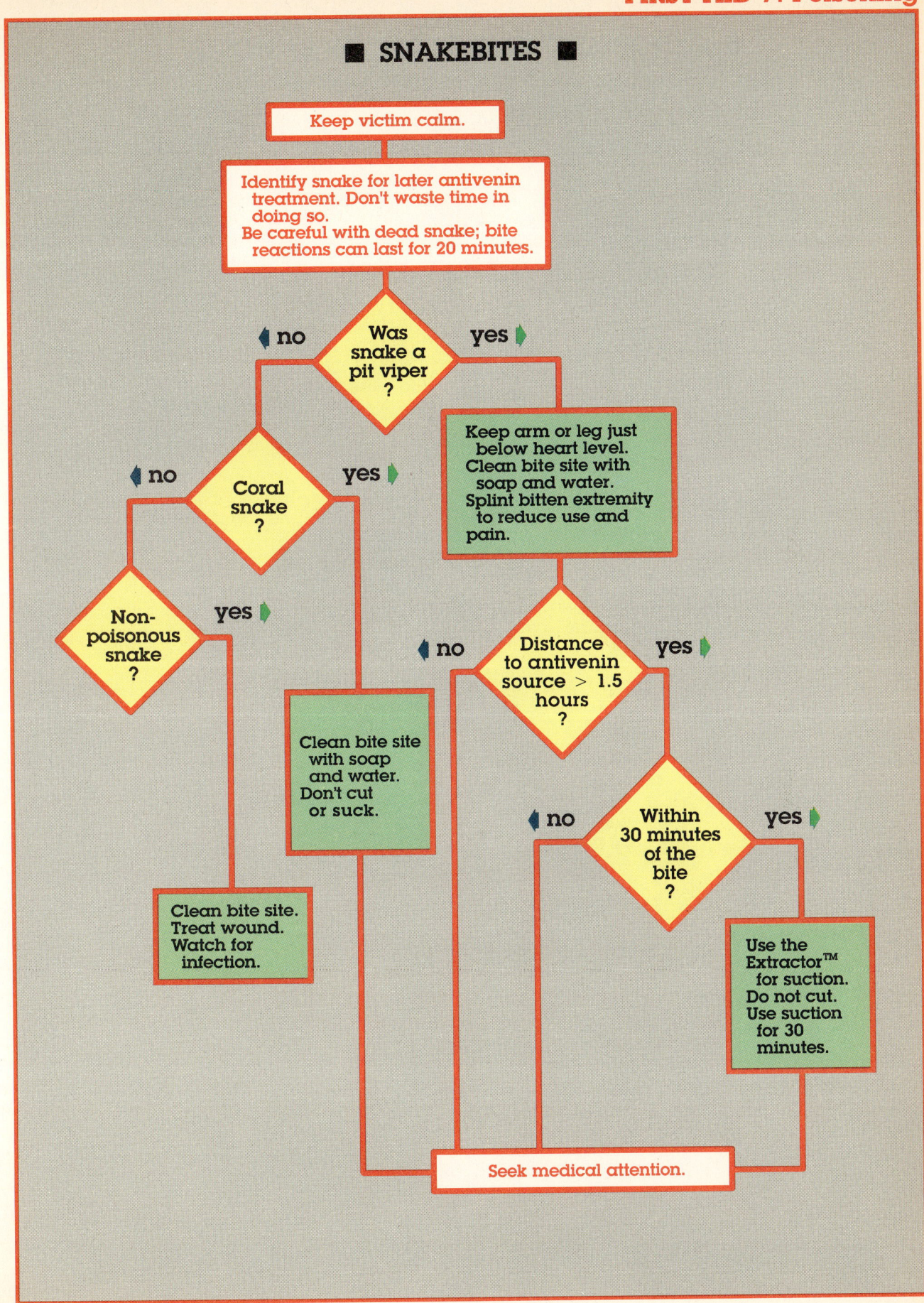

FIRST AID 7: Poisoning

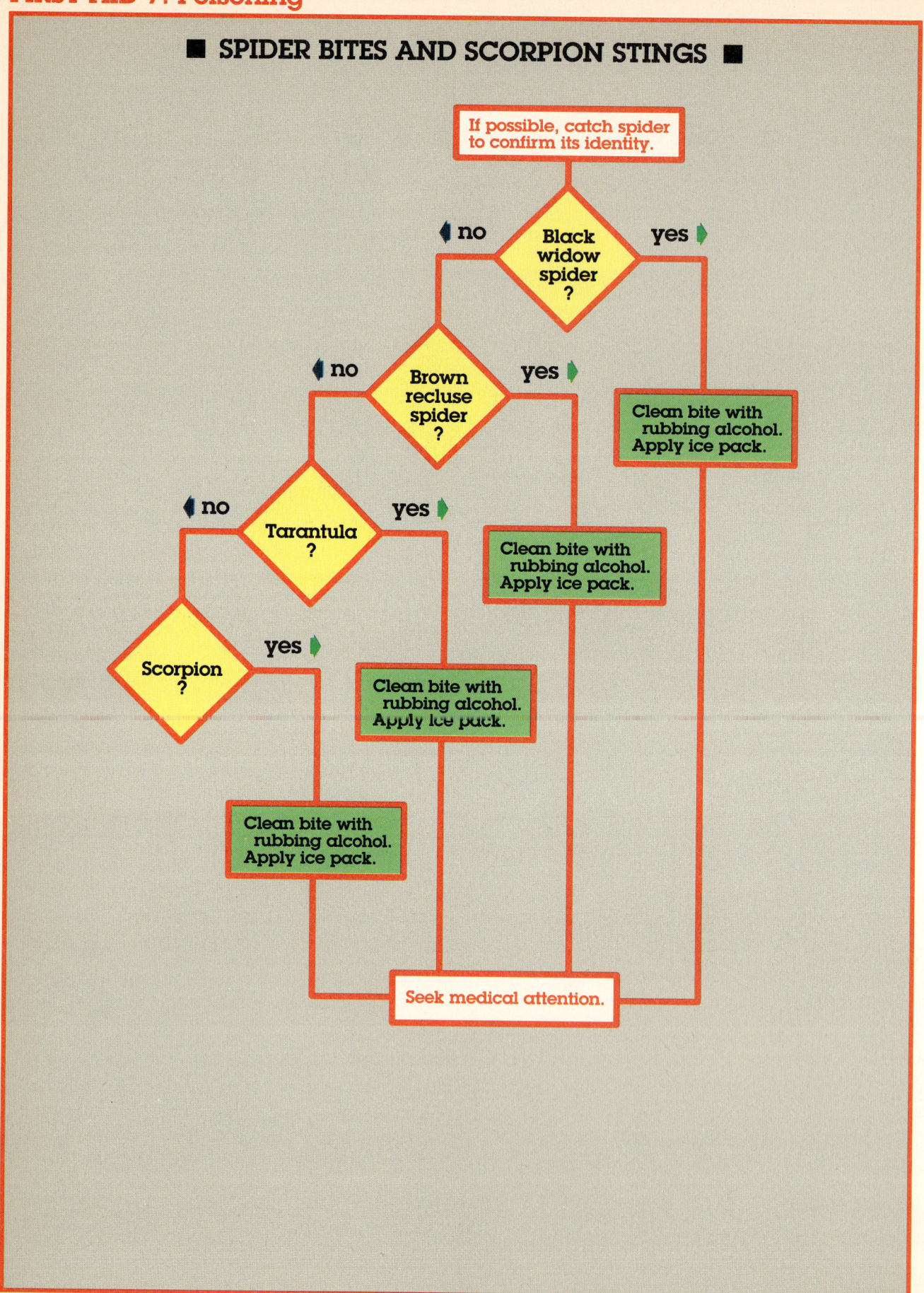

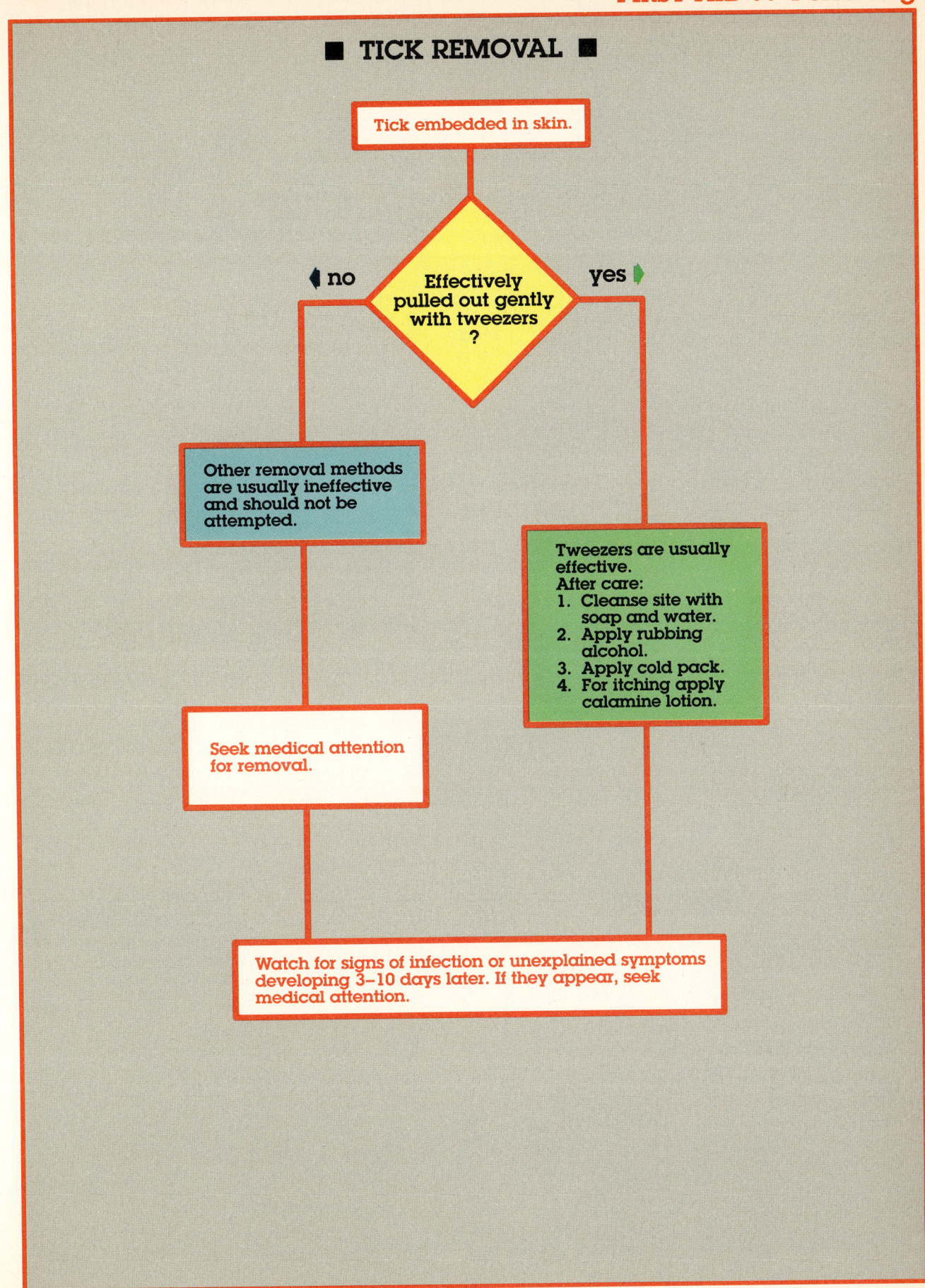

FIRST AID 7: Poisoning

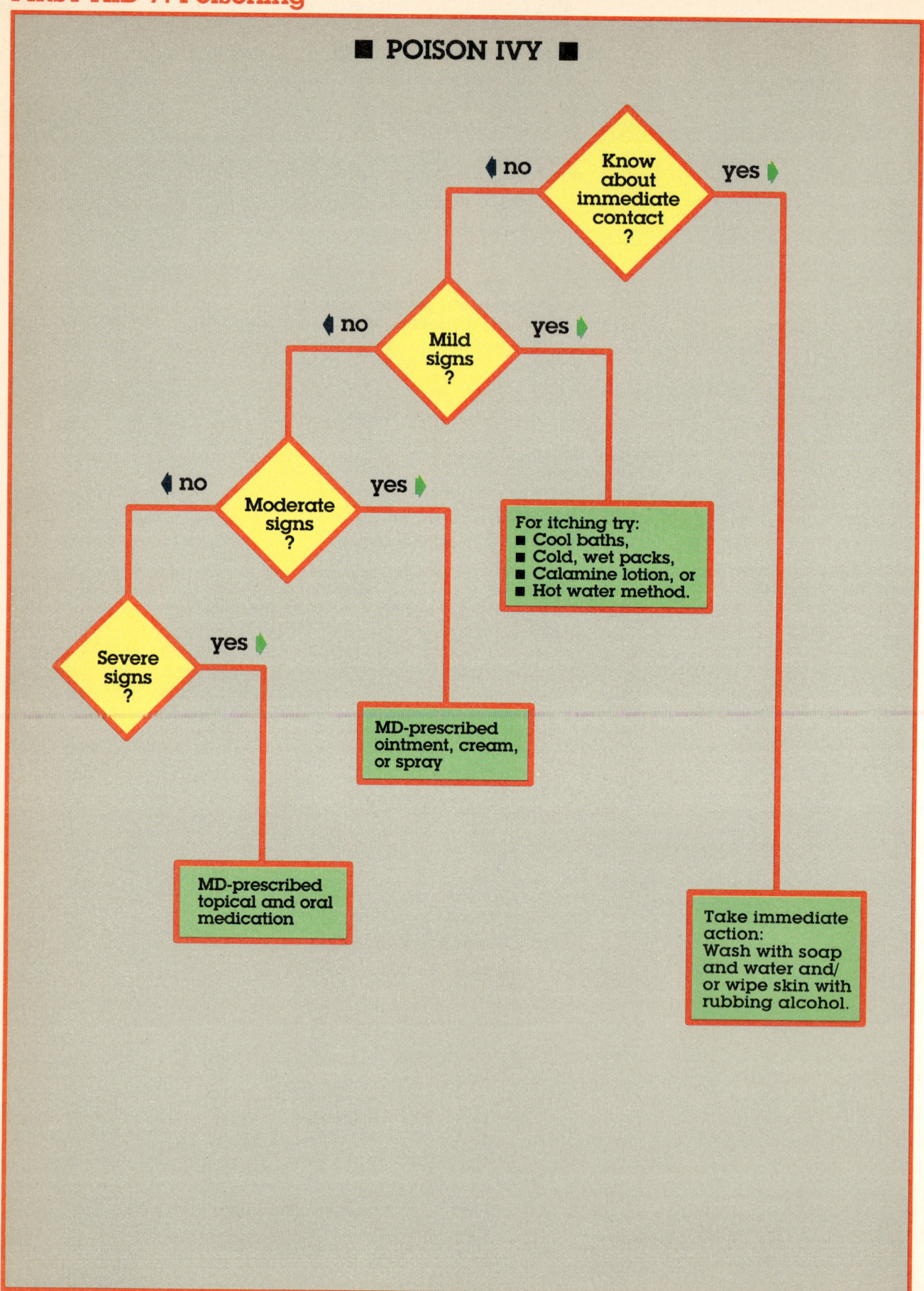

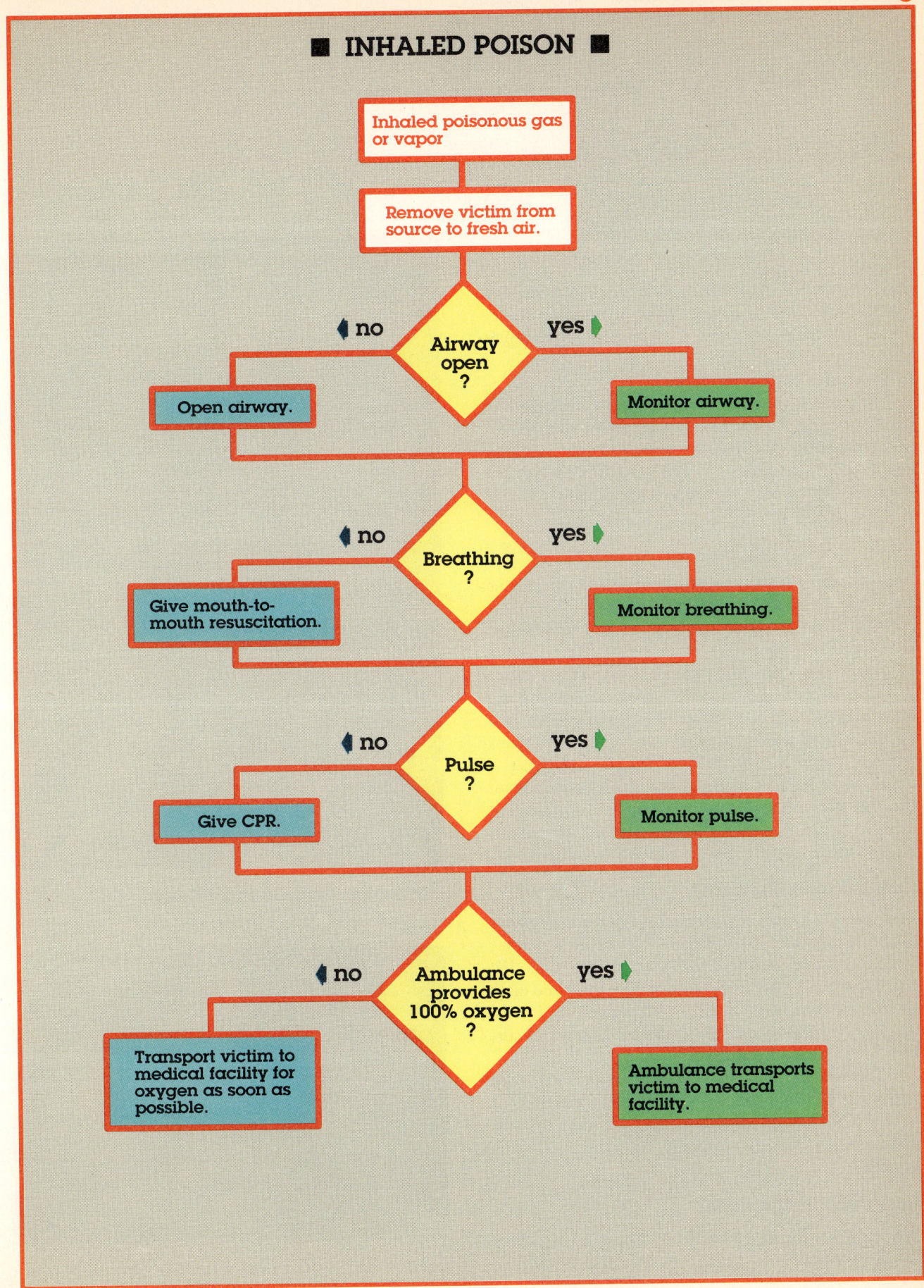

8 Burns

Heat Burns

More than two million burn injuries each year require medical attention or restriction of activity. Of these, about one-third are treated at hospital emergency departments. More than 6,000 persons die annually from injuries caused by burns.

The skin is sensitive to heat. Skin damage usually does not occur below 111 degrees Fahrenheit. Temperatures between 111 degrees and 123 degrees cause significant tissue damage. Temperatures above 123 degrees destroy skin within a brief moment.

Assessing a Burn

Assess a burn after any breathing or bleeding problems have been treated.

Controversy about whether or not first aiders should perform a burn assessment exists. Some authorities agree that it may be difficult to accurately determine the percentage and depth of a burn during the initial stages. They contend that such estimates are better done after waiting several days when the tissues become more clearly defined. On the other hand, many other experts contend that while that may be true, an attempt should be made since it is important to have an assessment for proper first aid. Therefore, a rapid but complete assessment is recommended.

How large is the burn?

The extent of a burn is expressed as a percentage of the total body surface. The familiar "Rule of Nines" defines a hand and arm as 9% of the body surface. Each leg counts as 18% of the body surface. The front and back torso are each valued at 18% with the genital area at 1%. The victim's hand size is about 1% and this surface area can be used for calculating most burns.

The Rule of Nines is accurate for adults, but it does not make allowances for the different proportions of a child. In small children the head accounts for 18% and each leg 14%. Accordingly, the Rule of Nines is modified.

How deep is the burn?

First-degree burns (superficial). These burns affect the skin's outer layer. Characteristics include redness,

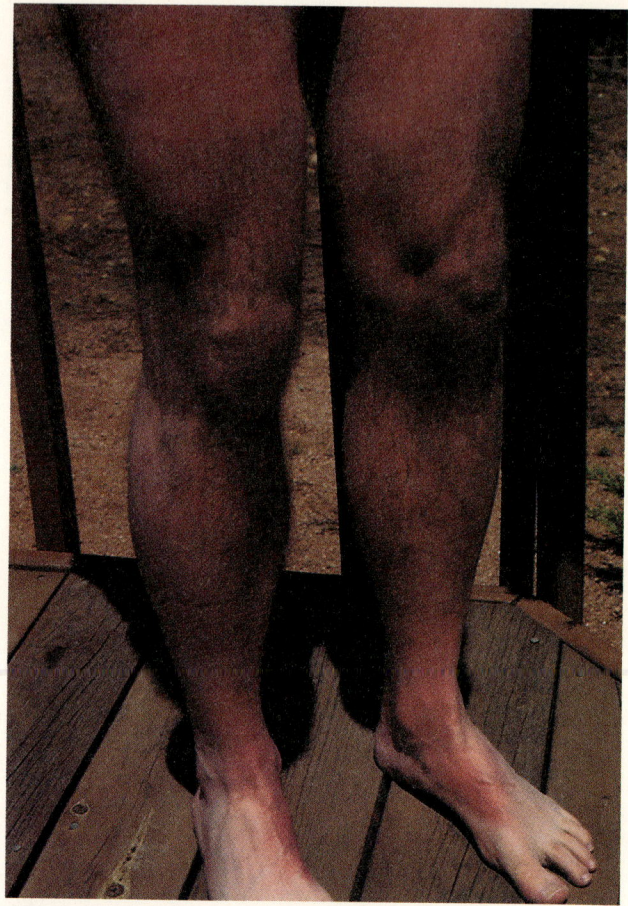

First-degree burn—sunburned legs

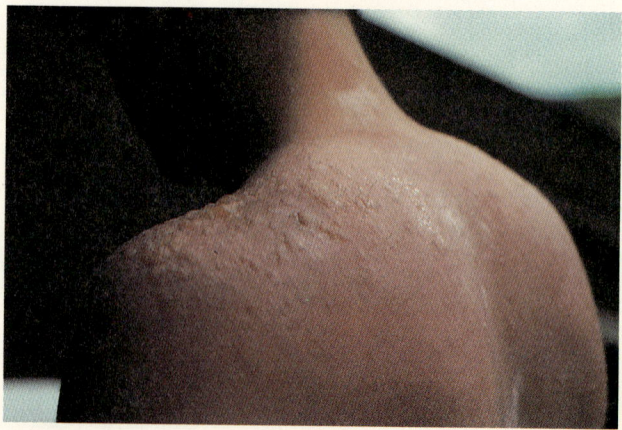

Second-degree burn—blistered shoulders

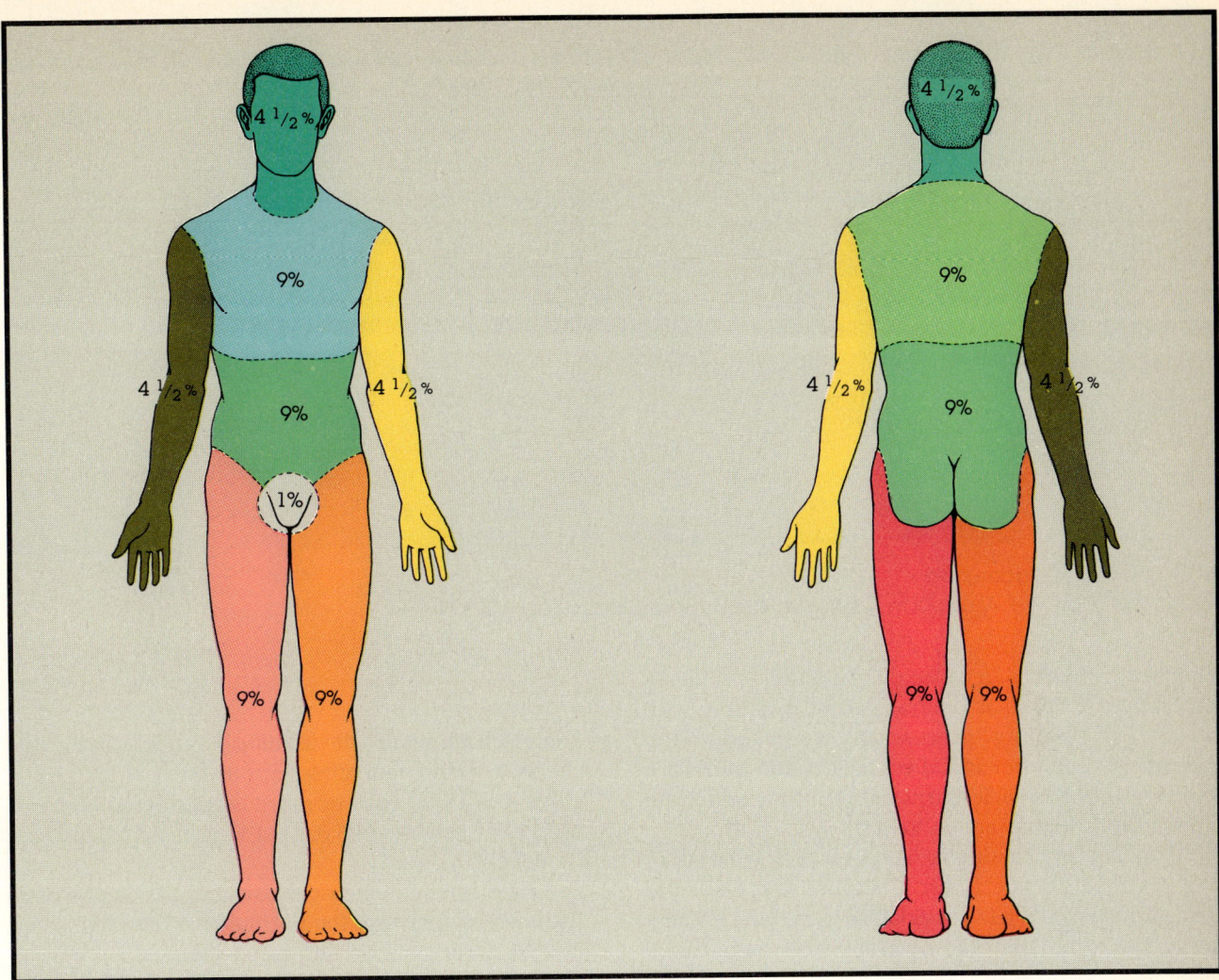

The "Rule of Nines"

mild swelling, tenderness, and pain. Healing occurs without scarring within a week.

Second-degree burns (partial-thickness). These burns extend through the entire outer skin layer and into the inner skin layer. Blister formation, swelling, weeping of fluids, and severe pain characterize second-degree burns. Intact blisters maintain a sterile covering whereas a broken blister results in a weeping wound.

Third-degree burns (full-thickness). These severe burns extend through all skin layers and into the underlying fat, muscle, and bone. Discoloration (charred, white, or cherry red), and a leathery, parchment-like, dry appearance indicate this degree of burn. Pain is absent because the nerve endings have been destroyed. Any pain found with this burn is caused by accompanying burns of lesser degrees (first- and second-degree). Proper healing requires skin grafting.

What parts of the body are burned?

Areas of most importance are the face (especially the eyelids), the hands, the feet, and the genitals. Respiratory tract burns are especially serious if associated with inhalation of fumes or heat.

How old is the burned victim?

A burn is considered more serious in an infant and in an elderly person (over 65) than in other victims.

Does the victim have any injuries or medical problems?

Burns can aggravate diabetes, heart disease, and lung disease, as well as other medical problems.

With this information and Table 8.1, the burn's severity can be determined as minor, moderate, or major (critical). Table 8.2 gives first aid for burns.

Chemical Burns

At least 25,000 products found in industry, agriculture, and the home can burn and cause tissue damage. A

TABLE 8-1 Burn Severity

Burn classification	Characteristics	
Minor burn	first-degree burn	
	second-degree burn	<15% BSA adults
	second-degree burn	<5% BSA in children/elderly persons
	third-degree burn	<2% BSA
Moderate burn	second-degree burn	15%–25% BSA in adults
	second-degree burn	10%–20% BSA in children/elderly persons
	third-degree burn	<10% BSA
Critical burn	second-degree burn	>25% BSA in adults
	second-degree burn	>20% BSA in children/elderly persons
	third-degree burn	>10% BSA
		Burns of hands, face, eyes, feet, or perineum
		Most victims with inhalation injury, electrical injury, major trauma, or significant preexisting diseases

BSA = Body surface area
Adapted from the American Burn Association categorization.

chemical continues to cause damage until it is inactivated by the tissue, is neutralized, or is diluted with water. The "burning" process may continue for long periods of time after initial contact. Alkali burns are more serious than acid burns because they penetrate deeper and remain active longer.

Toxicology training is not needed to treat all of the common chemical burns, because first aid is the same for all except a few special burns for which something has to be added to neutralize the chemical

Electrical Burns

Electrical injuries are devastating. Even with just a mild shock, a victim can suffer serious internal injuries. A current of 1,000 volts or more is considered high voltage, but even the 110 volts of household current can be deadly.

High voltage electrical currents passing through the body may disrupt the normal heart rhythm, cause cardiac arrest, burns, and other injuries.

TABLE 8-2 First Aid for Burns

Burn	Do	Don't
First-degree (redness, mild swelling, and pain)	Apply cold water and/or dry sterile dressing.	Apply butter, oleomargarine, etc.
Second-degree (deeper; blisters develop)	Immerse in cold water, blot dry with sterile cloth for protection. Treat for shock. Obtain medical attention if severe.	Break blisters. Remove shreds of tissue. Use antiseptic preparation, ointment spray, or home remedy on severe burn.
Third-degree (deeper destruction, skin layers destroyed)	Cover with sterile cloth to protect. Treat for shock. Watch for breathing difficulty. Obtain medical attention quickly.	Remove charred clothing that is stuck to burn. Apply ice. Use home medication.
Chemical Burn	Remove by flushing with large quantities of water for at least 15 minutes. Remove surrounding clothing. Obtain medical attention.	Neutralize

Source: U.S. Coast Guard.

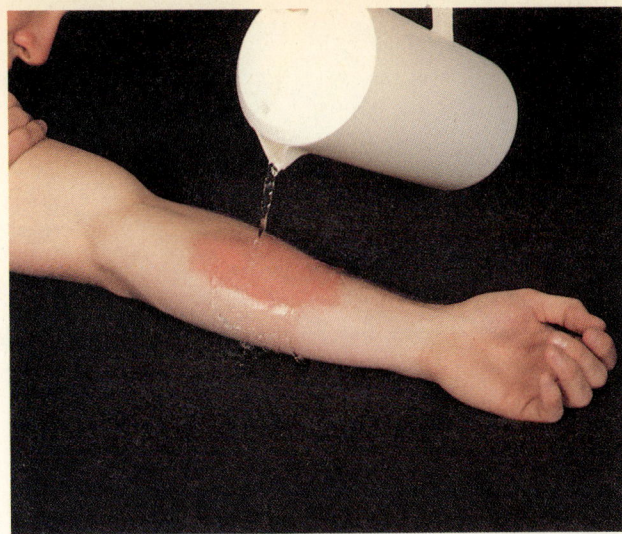
Washing/flooding chemical burn

When someone is electrocuted, electricity enters the body at the point of contact and travels along the path of least resistance (nerves and blood vessels). The current travels rapidly, generating heat and causing destruction. Usually, the electricity exits where the body is touching a surface or is in contact with a ground (e.g., a metal object). Sometimes, a victim may have more than one exit site.

Contact with Power Line (Outside Situations)

If electrocution comes from contact with a downed power line, the power must be turned off before a rescuer approaches anyone who may be in contact with the wire.

If the victim is in a car with a power line fallen across it, tell him or her to stay in the car until the power can be shut off. The only exception to this rule is when fire threatens the car. In this case, tell the victim to jump out of the car without making contact with the car or wire.

If you approach a victim and you feel a tingling sensation in your legs and lower body, stop. This sensation signals you are on energized ground and that an electrical current is entering through one foot, passing through your lower body, and leaving through the other foot. If this happens, raise a foot off the ground, turn around, and hop to a safe place.

If you can safely reach the victim, do *not* attempt to move any wires with wood poles, tools with wood handles, or objects with a high moisture content. Do *not* attempt to move downed wires at all unless you are trained and equipped with tools able to handle the high voltage.

Wait until the power company can cut the wires or disconnect them. Prevent bystanders from entering the danger area.

Contact Inside Buildings

Most electrical burns inside occur from faulty electrical equipment or careless use of electrical appliances. Turn off the electricity at the circuit breaker, fuse box, outside switch box, or unplug the appliance if the plug is undamaged. Do *not* touch the appliance or the victim until the current is off.

FIRST AID 8: Burns

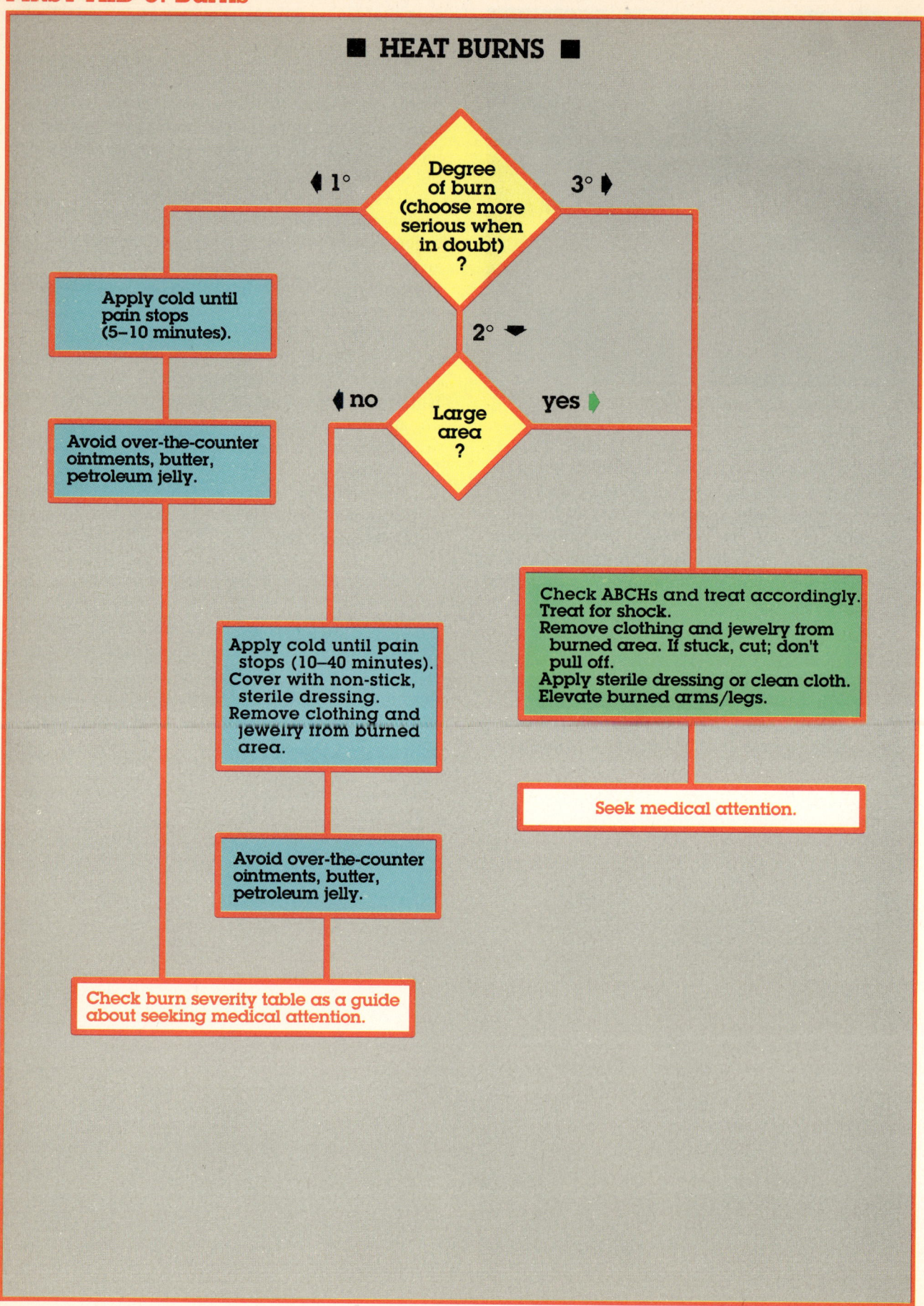

FIRST AID 8: Burns

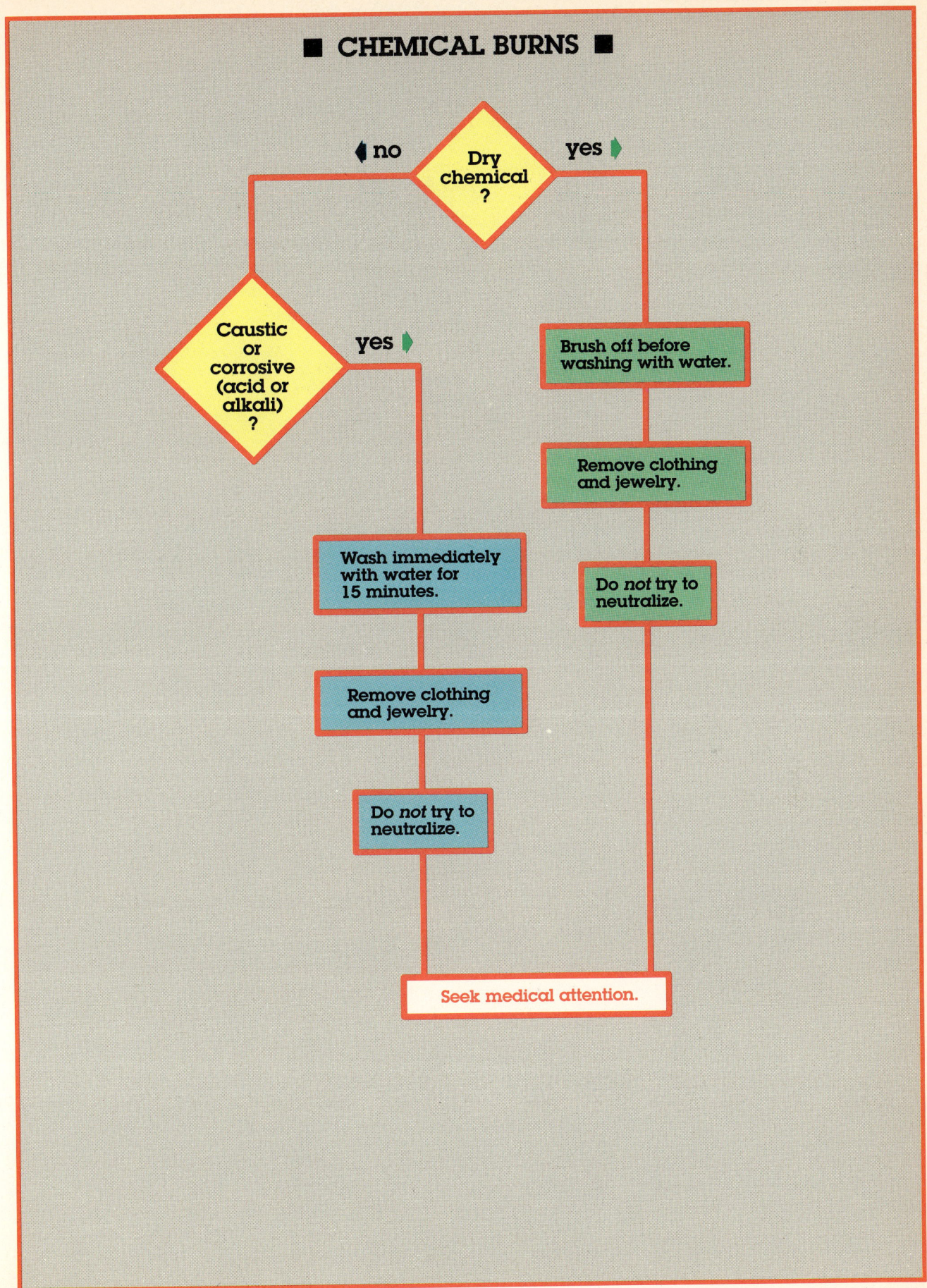

FIRST AID 8: Burns

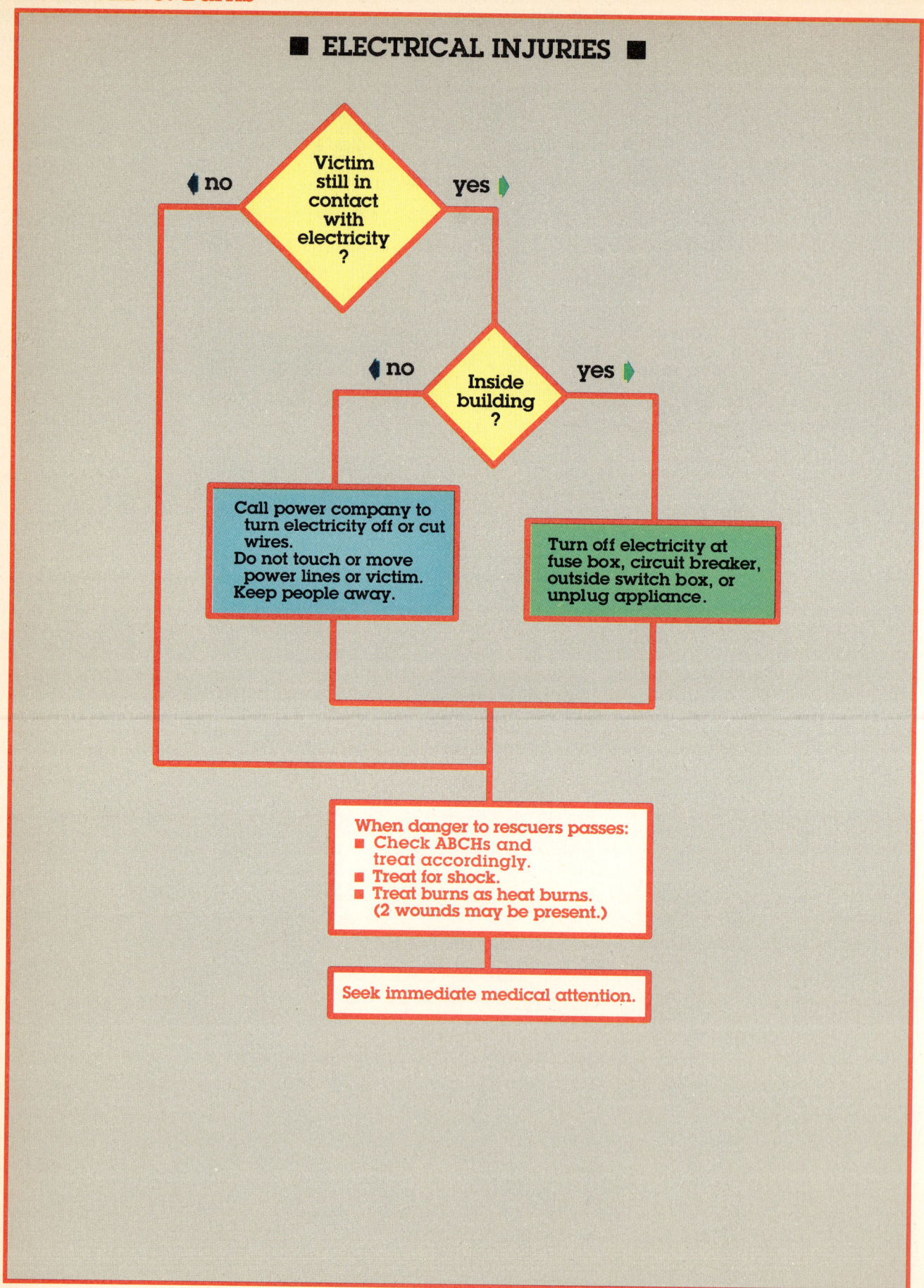

9

Cold- and Heat-Related Emergencies

Cold-Related Emergencies*

Frostbite

Frostbite occurs when temperatures drop below freezing. Tissue is damaged in two ways: (1) actual tissue freezing, which results in the formation of ice crystals between the tissue cells; the ice crystals enlarge by extracting water from the cells; and (2) the blood supply to the tissues is obstructed; this causes "sludged" blood clots, which prevent blood from flowing to the tissues. The second way injures more than the freezing does.

Frostbite mainly affects the feet, hands, ears, and nose. These areas do not contain large heat-producing muscles and are some distance from the heat generation sources. Moreover, when the body conserves heat, the blood supply diminishes in these areas first. The most severe consequences of frostbite are gangrene and amputation.

Some people are more prone to frostbite than others. Victims may also suffer from hypothermia.

Frostnip happens after long cold exposure but is not a serious problem. The condition is not usually painful. The skin becomes white or pale. First aid for frostnip consists of gently warming the affected area. This can be done with bare hands or by blowing warm air on the area.

Signs and Symptoms (Classified by Thawing)

Types (Based on the Pre-thaw Stage)

Superficial
- Skin color is white or grayish-yellow.
- Pain may occur early and later subside.
- Affected part may feel only very cold and numb. There may be a tingling, stinging, or aching sensation.
- Skin surface will feel hard or crusty and underlying tissue soft when depressed gently and firmly.

Deep
- Affected part feels hard, solid, and cannot be depressed.
- Blisters appear in 12 to 36 hours.

Source: National Ski Patrol protocols; adapted with permission.

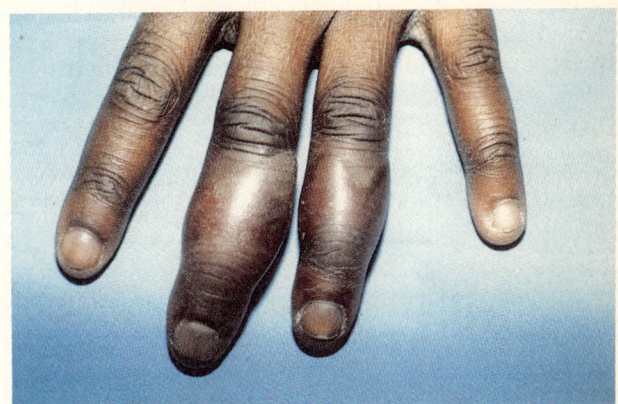

Frostbitten fingers, 6 hours after rewarming in 108°F water

- Affected part is cold with pale, waxy skin.
- A painfully cold part suddenly stops hurting.

Types (Based on the Post-thaw Stage)

After a part has thawed, frostbite can be categorized into degrees similar to the classification of burns. First-degree frostbite is superficial, while the other three are degrees of deep frostbite.

- ***First-degree frostbite.*** Affected part is warm, swollen, and tender.
- ***Second-degree frostbite.*** Blisters form within minutes to hours after thawing and enlarge over several days.
- ***Third-degree frostbite.*** Blisters are small, contain reddish-blue or purplish fluid. Surrounding skin may have a red or blue color and may not blanch when pressure is applied.
- ***Fourth-degree frostbite.*** No blisters or swelling occurs. The part remains numb, cold, white-to-dark purple in color.

All frostbite injuries follow the same first aid treatment. Seek medical attention immediately. **Rewarming of frostbitten parts seldom takes place outside of a medical facility.**

Hypothermia

Hypothermia results from a cooling of the body's core temperature. Hypothermia can occur at temperatures above freezing as well as below it. The victim may

65

suffer frostbite as well, if the body loses more heat than it produces. If the body temperature falls to 80°F, most people die. Hypothermia is not caused by outdoor exposure alone. It can also occur as a result of cool indoor temperatures. Death from hypothermia ranges from 20 to 85%.

Types of Hypothermia

A victim's core body temperature determines the type of hypothermia. To take the temperature, you need a low-reading thermometer, not the standard rectal thermometer, which is calibrated from 94 to 108°F. The recommended type is a rectal thermometer capable of reading temperatures between 84 to 108°F. These thermometers are uncommon.

1. *Mild* (above 90°F). Shivering, slurred speech, memory lapses, and fumbling hands. Victims frequently stumble and stagger. They are usually conscious and can talk. While many people suffer cold hands and feet, victims of mild hypothermia experience cold abdomens and backs, too.

2. *Profound* (below 90°F). Shivering has stopped. Muscles may become stiff and rigid, similar to rigor mortis. The victim's skin has a blue appearance and doesn't respond to pain; pulse and respirations slow down, and pupils dilate. The victim appears to be dead. Fifty to 80% of profound hypothermic victims die.

Heat-Related Emergencies

There are two types of major heat illness—heat stroke and heat exhaustion, and two types of minor heat illness—heat cramps and heat syncope. Table 9.1 describes the first three heat-related emergencies.

Heat Stroke (sunstroke)

Heat stroke is the most dangerous heat-related emergency. The death rate from this condition approaches 50%, even with appropriate medical care. Untreated victims always die. Heat stroke happens when the body is subjected to more heat than it can handle.

Types

- *Classic.* This type affects the elderly, chronically ill, obese, alcoholic, diabetic, and those with circulatory problems. It results from a combination of a hot environment and body mechanisms incapable of handling heat exposure.

TABLE 9-1 Heat-Related Emergencies

Indicators	Heat Cramps (least serious)	Heat Exhaustion (serious)	Heat Stroke (most serious)
Muscle cramps	Yes	No	No
Skin	Normal, moist-warm	Cold, clammy	Hot, dry
Temperature	Normal	Normal or slightly elevated	>105°F.
Loss of consciousness	Seldom	Sometimes	Usually
Perspiration	Heavy	Heavy	Little or none
First aid	Move to cool place.	Move to cool place.	Move to cool place.
	Rest affected muscle.	Elevate legs.	Elevate head and shoulders.
	Give a lot of cold water.	Cool victim.	Immediately cool victim.
	Do *not* massage.	If no improvement in 30 minutes, seek medical attention.	Immediately transport to medical facility.
			Monitor ABCs.
			Heat stroke is life-threatening!

- *Exertional.* This type affects a healthy individual when strenuously working or playing in a warm environment.

Signs and Symptoms

- Loss of consciousness
- Hot skin. Victims do not sweat because the sweating mechanism is overwhelmed. Half the victims with exertional heat stroke may have sweat on the skin since they are progressing from heat exhaustion (having sweaty skin) into heat stroke.
- High body temperature
- Rapid pulse and breathing
- Weakness, dizziness, headache

Heat Exhaustion

Heat exhaustion results from either excessive perspiration or the inadequate replacement of water lost by sweating. It is less critical than heat stroke, but it requires prompt attention because it can progress to heat stroke if left untreated.

Signs and Symptoms

- Heavy sweating
- Weakness
- Fast pulse
- Normal body temperature
- Headache and dizziness
- Nausea and vomiting

Heat Cramps

Heat cramps are painful muscle spasms in the arms or legs. They may occur when an excessive amount of body fluid is lost through sweating. Controversy exists regarding what type of liquid to drink—plain water, a commercial sports drink, or a saltwater solution. The body loses more water than electrolytes (sodium, potassium, etc.) during exercise. Experts generally agree that the primary need for those sweating in hot environments is to replace the water lost from heavy sweating, rather than the electrolytes. However, mildly salted water (¼ to 1 level teaspoon in 1 quart of water) or electrolyte drink can be given.

Routine use of salt tablets to prevent heat cramps is no longer recommended since they can induce high blood pressure and hinder adjustment to heat.

Signs and Symptoms

- Severe cramping, usually affecting arms or legs
- Abdominal cramping

Heat Syncope

This condition resembles fainting and is usually self-correcting. Victims who are not nauseous can drink water. If no nausea and/or vomiting occurs, water can be given. First aid consists of having the victim lie down in a cool place.

FIRST AID 9: Cold- and Heat-Related Injuries

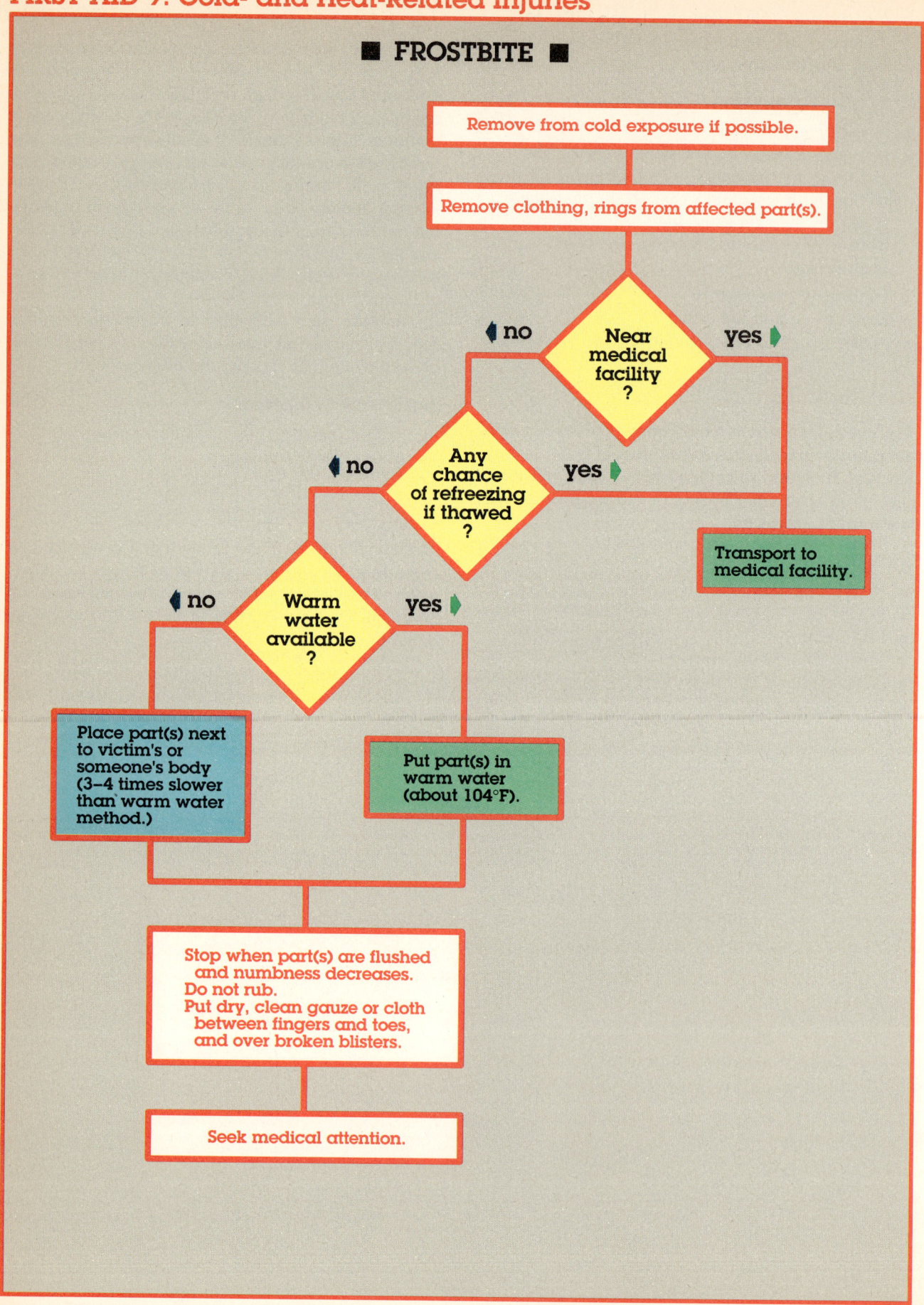

FIRST AID 9: Cold- and Heat-Related Injuries

■ HYPOTHERMIA ■

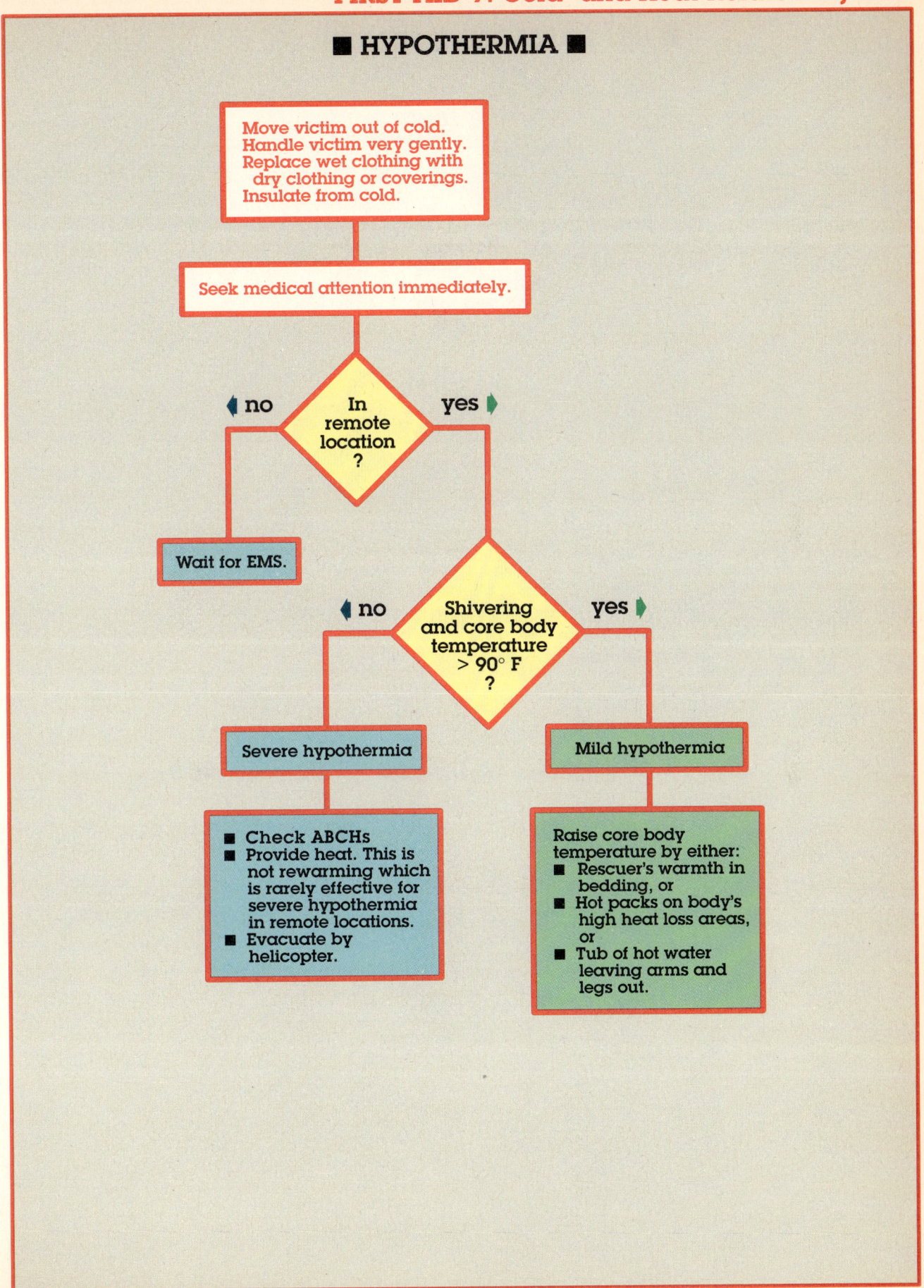

FIRST AID 9: Cold- and Heat-Related Injuries

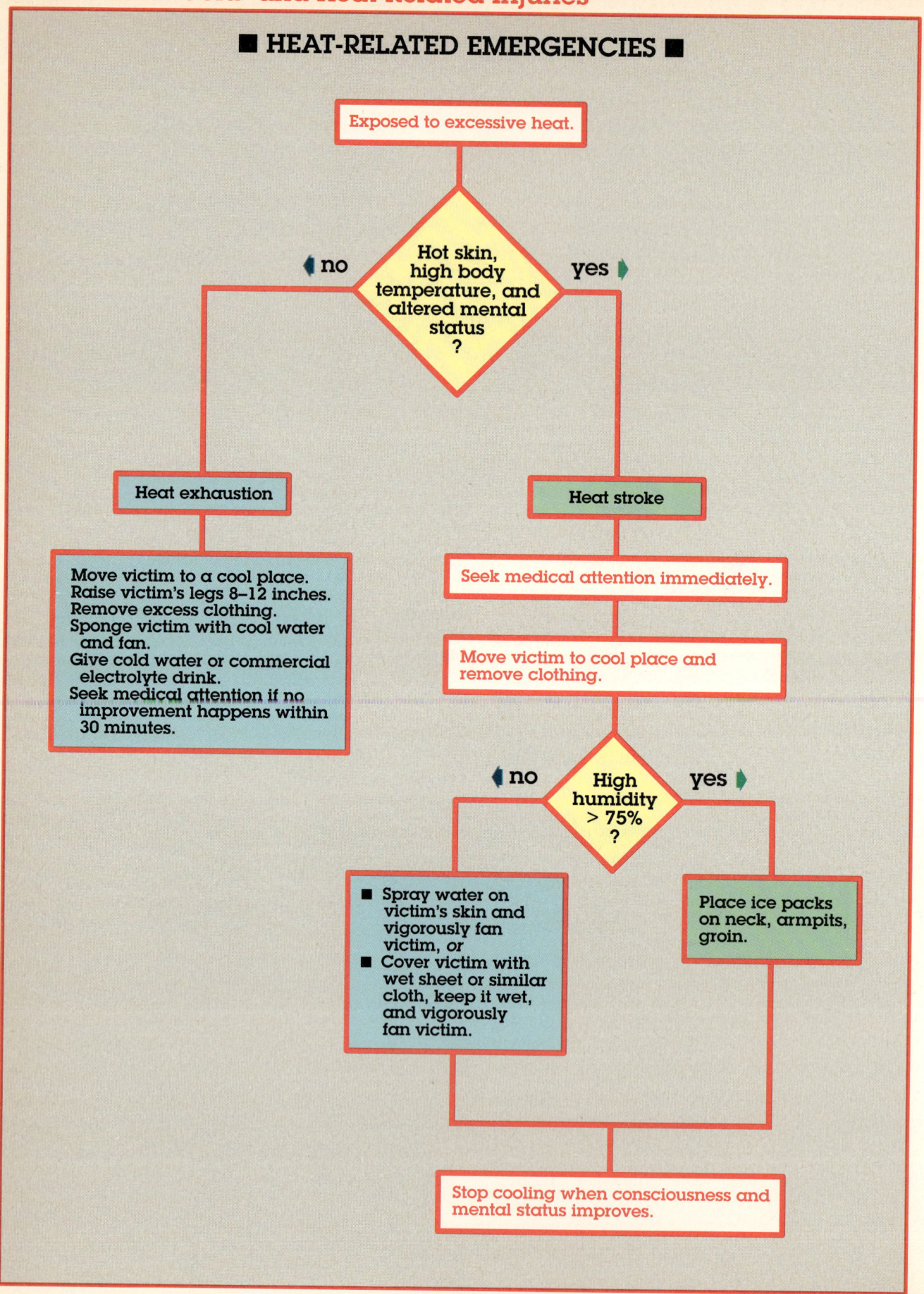

10
Bone, Joint, and Muscle Injuries*

Fractures

The terms **fracture** and **broken bone** have the same meaning—a break or crack in a bone. Fractures are classified as being **open** (when the skin is broken and bleeds externally) or **closed** (when the skin has not been broken).

Fracture Classification

- **Open (compound) fracture.** The overlaying skin has been damaged or broken. The wound can be produced either by the bone protruding through the skin or by a direct blow cutting the skin at the time of the fracture. The bone may not always be seen in the wound. Any broken bone which is covered by damaged skin is classified as an open fracture.
- **Closed (simple) fracture.** The skin has not been broken and no wound exists anywhere near the fracture site.

Open fractures are more serious than closed fractures because of greater blood loss and greater chance of infection.

Signs and Symptoms

- **Swelling.** Caused by bleeding; it occurs rapidly after a fracture.
- **Deformity.** This is not always obvious. Compare the injured with the uninjured opposite part when checking for deformity.
- **Pain and tenderness.** Commonly found only at the injury site. The victim will usually be able to point to the site of the pain. A useful procedure for detecting fractures is to gently feel along the bones; complaints about pain or tenderness serve as a reliable sign of a fracture.
- **Loss of use.** (Inability to use the injured part ("guarding"). Because motion produces pain, the victim will refuse to use it. However, sometimes the victim is able to move the limb with little or no pain.
- **Grating sensation.** Do *not* move the injured limb in an attempt to see if a grating sensation (called **crepitus**) can be felt and even sometimes heard when the broken bone ends rub together.
- **History of the injury.** suspect a fracture whenever severe accidents (e.g., motor-vehicle accidents and falls) happen. The victim may have heard or felt the bone snap.

Spinal Injuries

The spine is a column of vertebrae stacked one on the next from the skull's base to the tail bone. It encloses the spinal cord, which consists of long tracts of nerves that join the brain with all body organs and parts. It protects the spinal nerves.

If a broken spinal column pinches spinal nerves, paralysis can result. All unconscious victims should be treated as though they had spinal injuries. All conscious victims sustaining injuries from falls, diving accidents, auto accidents, or cave-in should be carefully checked for spine injuries before moving them.

A mistake in handling a spinal injured victim could mean a lifetime in a wheelchair or bed for the victim.

Signs and Symptoms

- Possible spinal injury in all severe accidents (e.g., motor-vehicle, falls, dives into water)
- Head injuries (They serve as a clue, since the head may have been snapped suddenly in one or more directions, endangering the spine. About 15% to 20% of head-injured victims also have neck and spinal cord injuries.)
- Painful movement of arms and/or legs
- Numbness, tingling, weakness, or burning sensation in arms or legs
- Loss of bowel or bladder control
- Paralysis to arms and/or legs
- Deformity (odd angle of the victim's head and neck)

Ask the conscious victim the following questions:

- **Is there pain?** Neck injuries (cervical) radiate pain to the arms; upper back injuries (thoracic) radiate pain around the ribs and into the chest; lower back injuries (lumbar) usually radiate pain down the legs. Often the victim describes the pain as "electric."

*Source: Based upon American Academy of Orthopaedic Surgeons protocols.

- **Can you move your feet?** Ask the victim to move his or her foot against your hand. If the victim cannot perform this movement or if the movement is extremely weak against your hand, the victim may have injured the cord.
- **Can you move your fingers?** Moving the fingers is a sign that nerve pathways are intact. Ask the victim to grip your hand. A strong grip indicates that a spinal cord injury is unlikely.

For an unconscious victim:

- Look for cuts, bruises, and deformities.
- Test responses by pinching the victim's hands (either palm or back) and feet (sole or top of the bare foot). No reaction could mean possible spinal cord damage.
- Ask others about what happened.

If not sure about a possible spinal injury, assume that the victim has one until proven otherwise.

Muscle Injuries

Though muscle injuries pose no real emergency, first aiders have ample opportunities to care for them.

Muscle Strains

A muscle strain, also known as muscle pull, occurs when the muscle is stretched beyond its normal range of motion, resulting in a muscle fiber tear. A range of severity exists.

Signs and Symptoms

- A sharp pain immediately after the injury
- Extreme tenderness when area is felt
- Disfigurement (indentation, cavity, or bump)
- Severe weakness and loss of function of the injured part
- The sound of a snap when the tissue is torn

Muscle Contusions

Muscle contusions result from a blow to a muscle. This injury is also known as a bruise.

Muscle Cramps

Muscles can go into an uncontrolled spasm and contraction, resulting in severe pain and a restriction or loss of movement. Some experts believe that diet or fluid loss explains muscle cramping. Nevertheless, many different things can cause muscle cramps; no one knows all the causes.

Cryotherapy

Ice is one of the most versatile treatments available for injuries. This form of treatment, called **cryotherapy,** uses ice or other cold applications for muscle strains, bruises, joint sprains, insect stings, and minor burns.

Reducing tissue temperature constricts blood vessels (helps by controlling bleeding), and reduces pain.

Forms of Ice Therapy

- *Ice massage.* Rubbing ice cubes in a circular motion on the affected area for 7 to 10 minutes on regions with little fat (e.g., elbow) and about 20 minutes in areas with more fat (e.g., leg muscles) is recommended.
- *Ice bags.* Apply a bag full of crushed ice or an ice cube to the affected area for 10 to 30 minutes. This method penetrates and lasts longer than the ice massage.
- *Cold water immersion.* An ice slush (ice cubes or crushed ice added to a bucket of water) is useful for injuries to the hand, foot, or elbow. Allow the injured part to soak in the ice slush for 10 to 20 minutes.
- *Cold packs.* Sealed plastic pouches containing a refreezable gel are available commercially. These can get very cold, so it is important that the cold packs be wrapped in a towel and that they never be applied directly to the skin.
- *Chemical "snap packs."* These sealed pouches resemble cold packs but contain two chemical envelopes that, when squeezed, mix the chemicals. A chemical reaction produces a cooling effect. Though they don't cool as well as other methods, snap packs are convenient.

Precautions include *NOT* exposing the skin to cold too long, which can result in frostbite. Those with any form of cold allergy, Raynaud's phenomenon, or abnormal sensitivity to cold should avoid cryotherapy.

Other tips when using ice or other forms of cryotherapy include the following:

- Apply ice or cold immediately after an injury.
- Raise the injured area above heart level.
- Apply ice or cold for no more than 30 minutes at a time. Repeat two to four times a day until fully recovered.

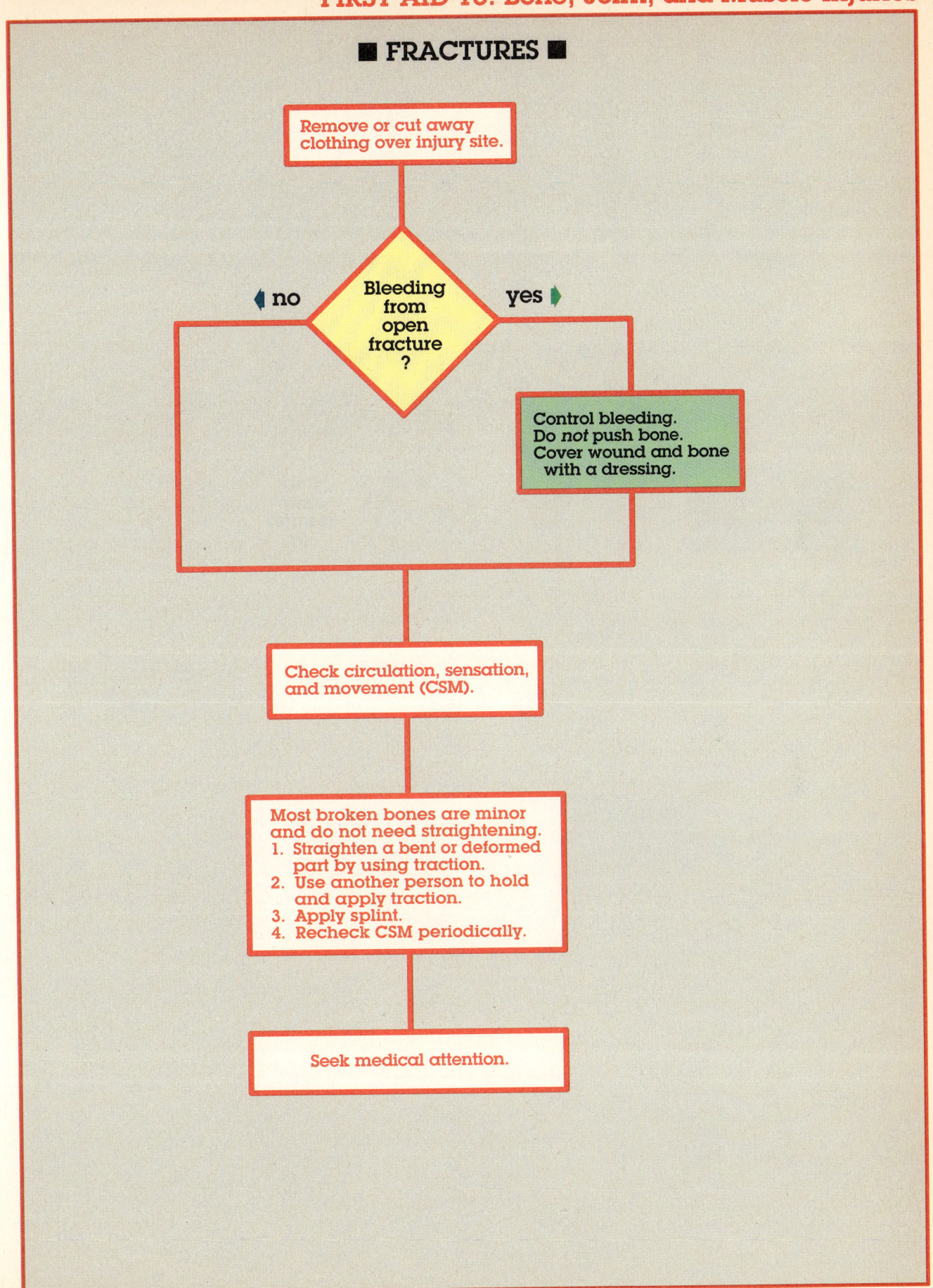

FIRST AID 10: Bone, Joint, and Muscle Injuries

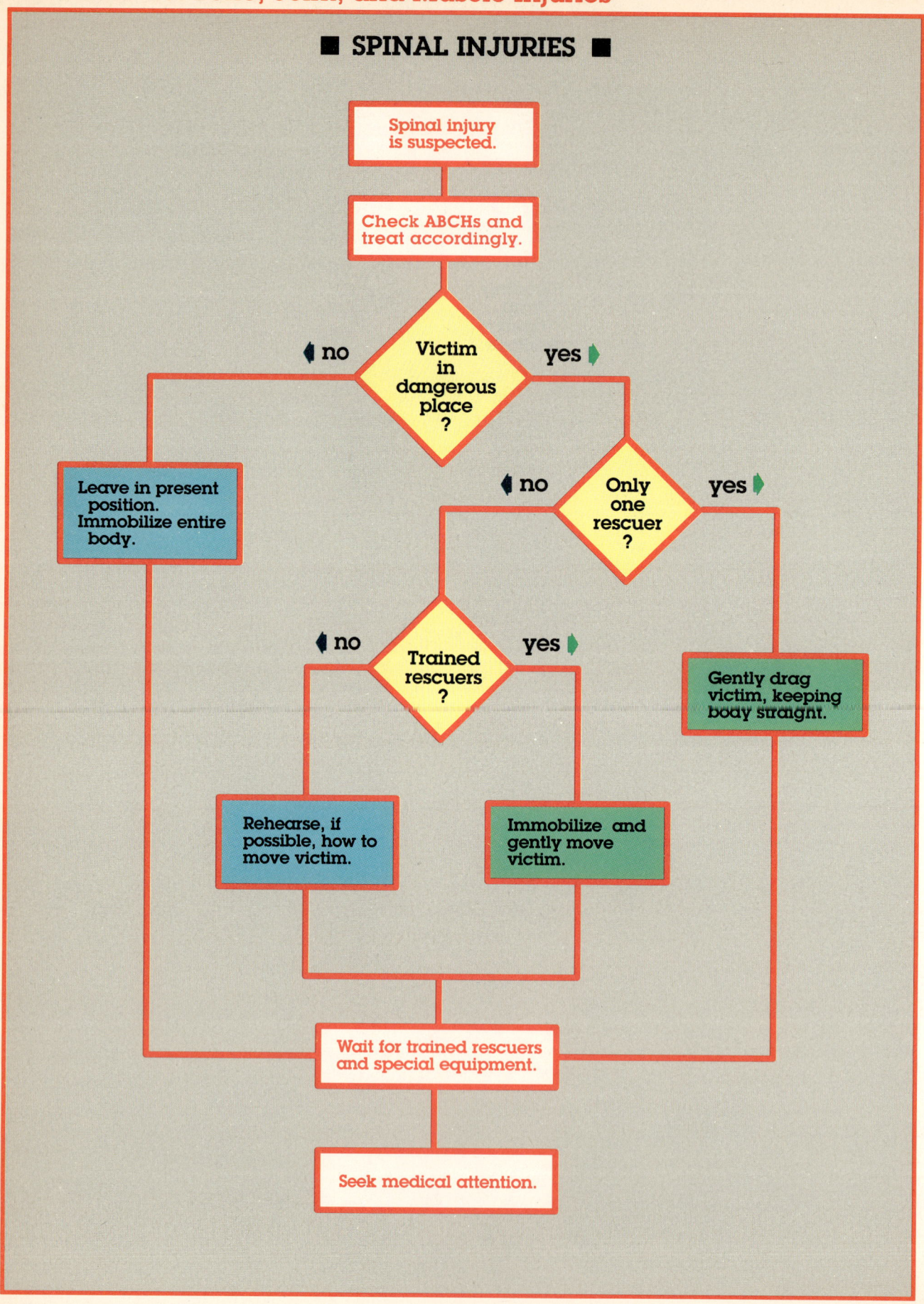

FIRST AID 10: Bone, Joint, and Muscle Injuries

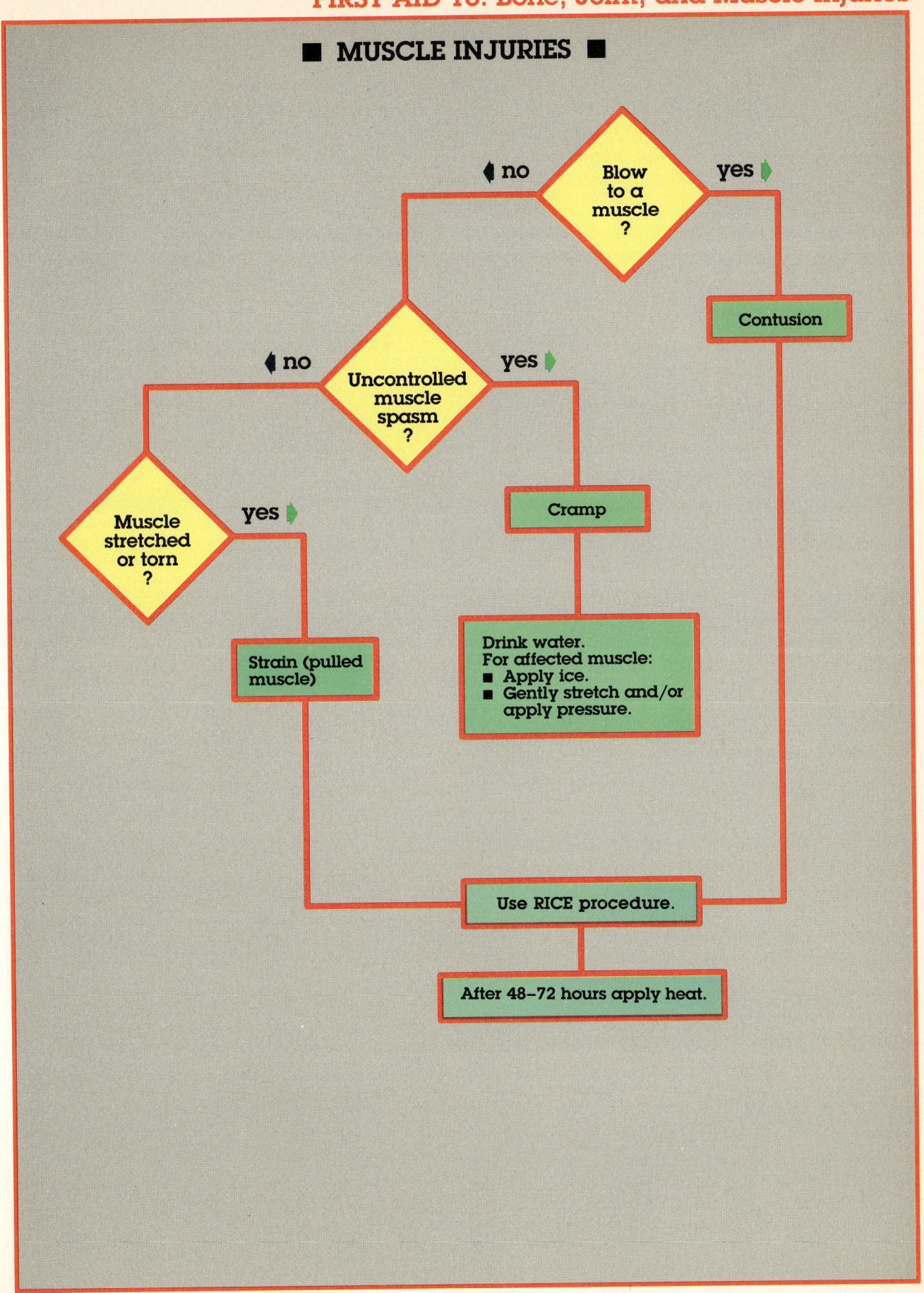

FIRST AID 10: Bone, Joint, and Muscle Injuries

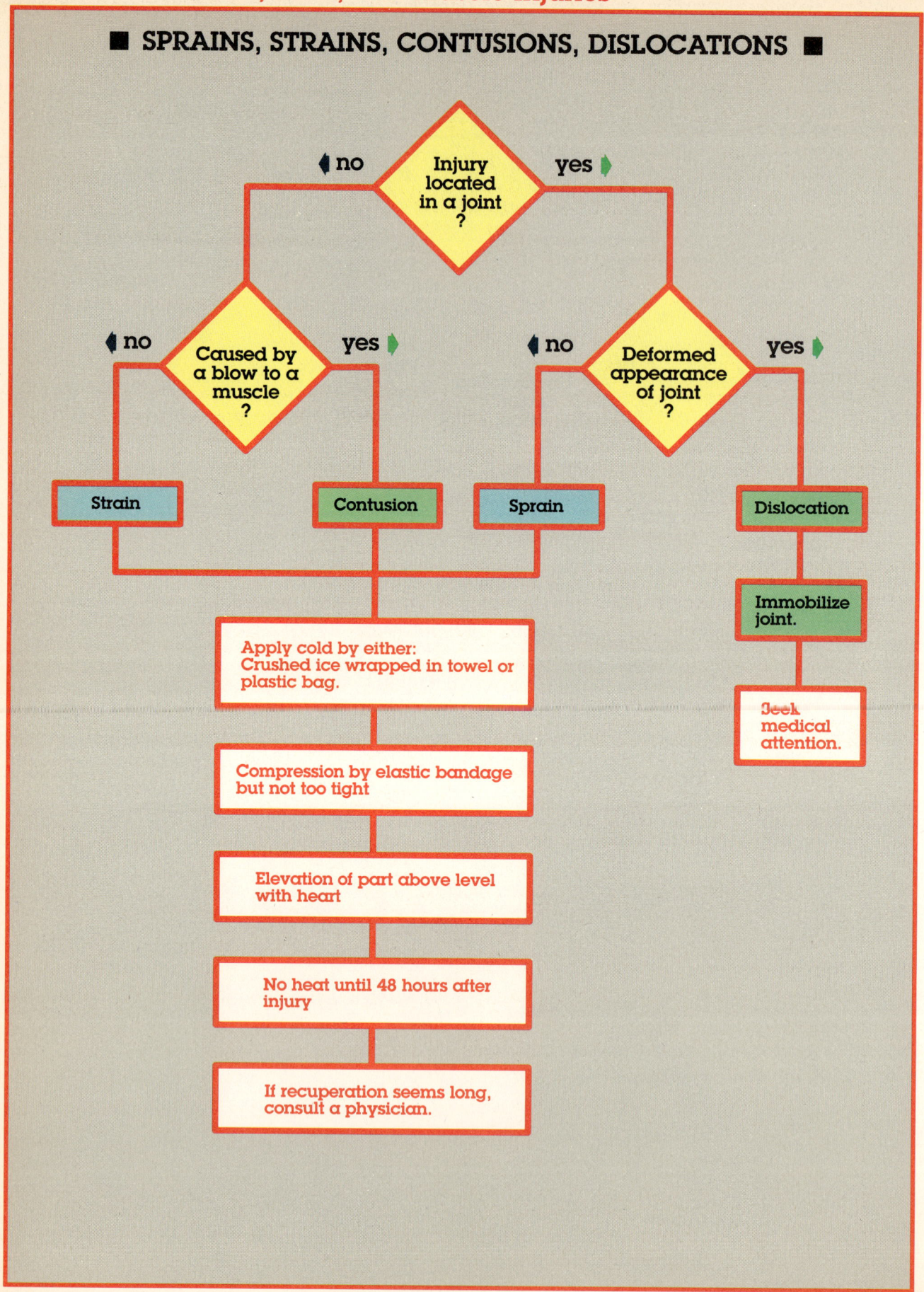

11
Medical Emergencies

Heart Attack*

A heart attack occurs when the blood supply to a part of the heart muscle is severely reduced or stopped because of an obstruction in one of the coronary arteries (these supply the heart with its blood). A buildup of fatty deposits along the coronary artery's inner wall is one reason for blood obstruction. The blood supply can also be reduced when the artery goes into a spasm.

Signs and Symptoms

Heart attacks are difficult to determine. Because medical care at the onset of a heart attack is vital to survival and the quality of recovery, the rule to follow is that if you suspect a heart attack for any reason, seek medical attention at once rather than delaying.

The American Heart Association lists these as possible signs and symptoms of a heart attack:

- Uncomfortable pressure, fullness, squeezing, or pain in the center of the chest, lasting two minutes or longer. It may come and go.
- Pain may spread to either shoulder, the neck, the lower jaw, or either arm.
- Any or all of the following: weakness, dizziness, sweating, nausea, or shortness of breath.

Not all of these warning signs occur in every heart attack. Many victims will deny that they might be having a heart attack. If you see some of these signs, however, don't delay seeking medical attention. Time loss can seriously increase the risk of major damage. Get help immediately!

Stroke*

A **stroke** is also known as a **cerebrovascular accident (CVA).** A stroke occurs when a blood vessel that is bringing oxygen and nutrients to the brain bursts or becomes clogged by a blood clot, preventing part of the brain from receiving the flow of blood it needs. Stroke is the third largest cause of death in America. It is also a major cause of disability.

Signs and Symptoms

Signs and symptoms of a stroke depend on the area of the brain involved:

- Sudden weakness or numbness of the face, arm, and leg on one side of the body
- Loss of speech, or trouble talking or understanding speech
- Dimness or loss of vision, particularly in only one eye; unequal pupils
- Unexplained dizziness, unsteadiness or sudden falls.
- Sudden severe headache
- Loss of bladder and/or bowel control

About 10% of strokes are preceded by "little strokes" (transient ischemic attacks, or TIAs). TIAs are extremely important warning signs for stroke. TIA symptoms are very similar to those of a full-fledged stroke. Do *not* ignore TIAs; get medical attention immediately.

Diabetic Emergencies*

Diabetes is the inability of the body to appropriately metabolize carbohydrates. The pancreas fails to produce enough of a hormone called insulin. The function of insulin is to take sugar from the blood and carry it into the cells to be used. When excess sugar remains in the blood, the body cells must rely on fat as fuel. Since blood sugar is a major body fuel, when it cannot be used, diabetes develops.

When the blood sugar level becomes too high because of too little insulin in the blood, diabetic coma, or **ketoacidosis,** may occur. Meanwhile, the cells, deprived of sugar, begin to use fats for fuel. Use of fat results in the production of acids and ketones as wastes. The ketones give the victims' breath a fruity odor.

The opposite condition, insulin shock, can result when a person with diabetes has taken too much insulin or has not eaten. The blood sugar level drops dangerously low and the victim becomes weak and disoriented, or unconscious.

Both of these conditions can be fatal unless something is done to reverse them.

Source: American Heart Association; adapted with permission.

Source: American Diabetes Association; reprinted with permission.

Epilepsy*

Types of Seizures

Epileptic seizures may be convulsive or nonconvulsive in nature, depending on where in the brain the malfunction takes place and on how much of the total brain area is involved.

Convulsive seizures are the ones that most people generally think of when they hear the word "epilepsy." In this type of seizure the person undergoes convulsions that usually last from two to five minutes, with complete loss of consciousness and muscle spasm.

Nonconvulsive seizures may take the form of a blank stare lasting only a few seconds, an involuntary movement of an arm or leg, or a period of automatic movement in which awareness of one's surroundings is blurred or completely absent.

Since these seizure types are so different, they require different kinds of action from a first aider, and some require no action at all.

An uncomplicated convulsive seizure due to epilepsy is not a medical emergency, even though it looks like one. After a few minutes, it stops naturally without ill effects. The average victim is able to resume normal activity after a rest period and may need only little or no assistance in getting home.

However, several medical conditions other than epilepsy can cause seizures. These require immediate medical attention and include:

encephalitis	pregnancy
meningitis	hypoglycemia
heat stroke	high fever
poisoning	head injury

The following guidelines are designed to help epileptics avoid unnecessary and expensive trips to the emergency room and to help you decide whether or not to call an ambulance when someone has a convulsive seizure.

Reasons to call the EMS system include:

- A seizure that lasts more than five minutes.
- There is no "epilepsy" or "seizure disorder" identification.
- Slow recovery, a second seizure, or difficult breathing afterwards.
- Pregnancy or other medical condition identification.
- Any signs of injury or illnesses.

The Epilepsy Foundation of America lists these first aid procedures for seizures (convulsions, generalized tonic-clonic, grand mal seizures):

1. Cushion the victim's head
2. Loosen the victim's tight neckwear
3. Turn the victim onto side
4. Look for a medic alert tag (bracelet or necklace)
5. As seizure ends, offer your help. Most seizures in people with epilepsy are not medical emergencies. They end after a minute or two without harm and usually do not require medical attention.

Precautions in caring for a seizure victim:

- Do *not* give anything to eat or drink.
- Do *not* hold the victim down.
- Do *not* put anything between the victim's teeth during the seizure.
- Do *not* throw any liquid on the victim's face or into his or her mouth.
- Do *not* embarass victim—clear away bystanders.

---

*Source: Epilepsy Foundation of America; reprinted with permission.

FIRST AID 11: Medical Emergencies

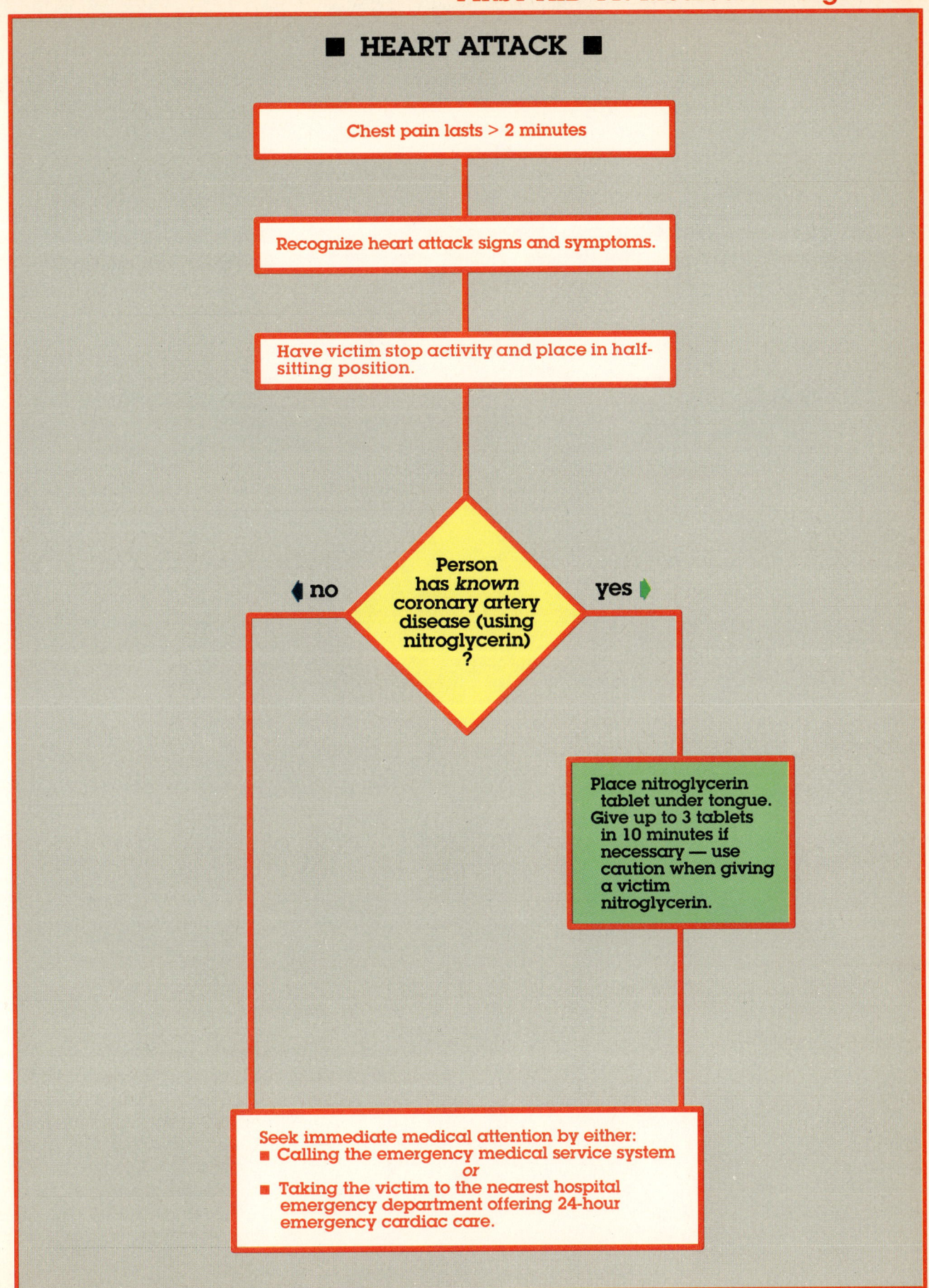

FIRST AID 11: Medical Emergencies

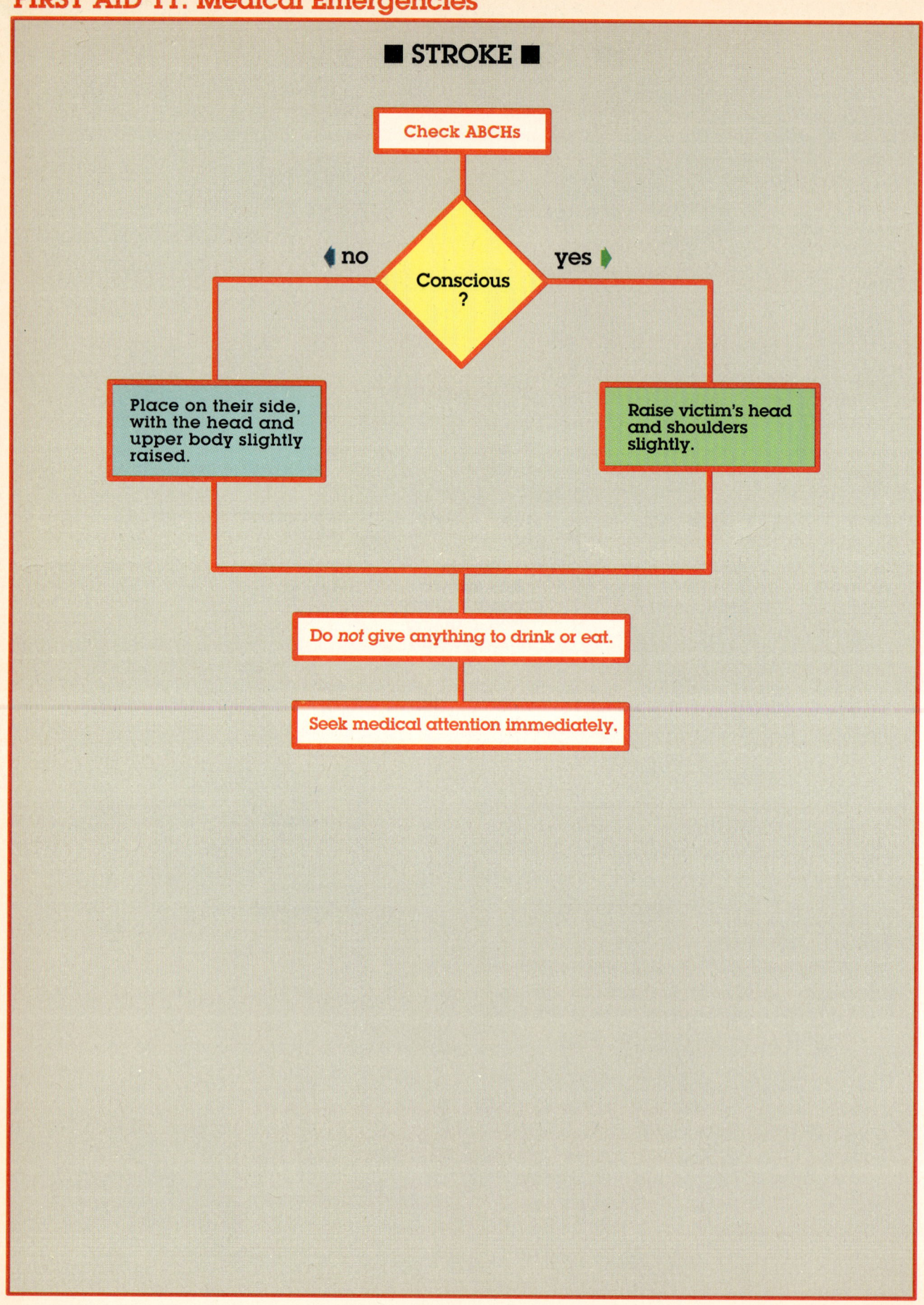

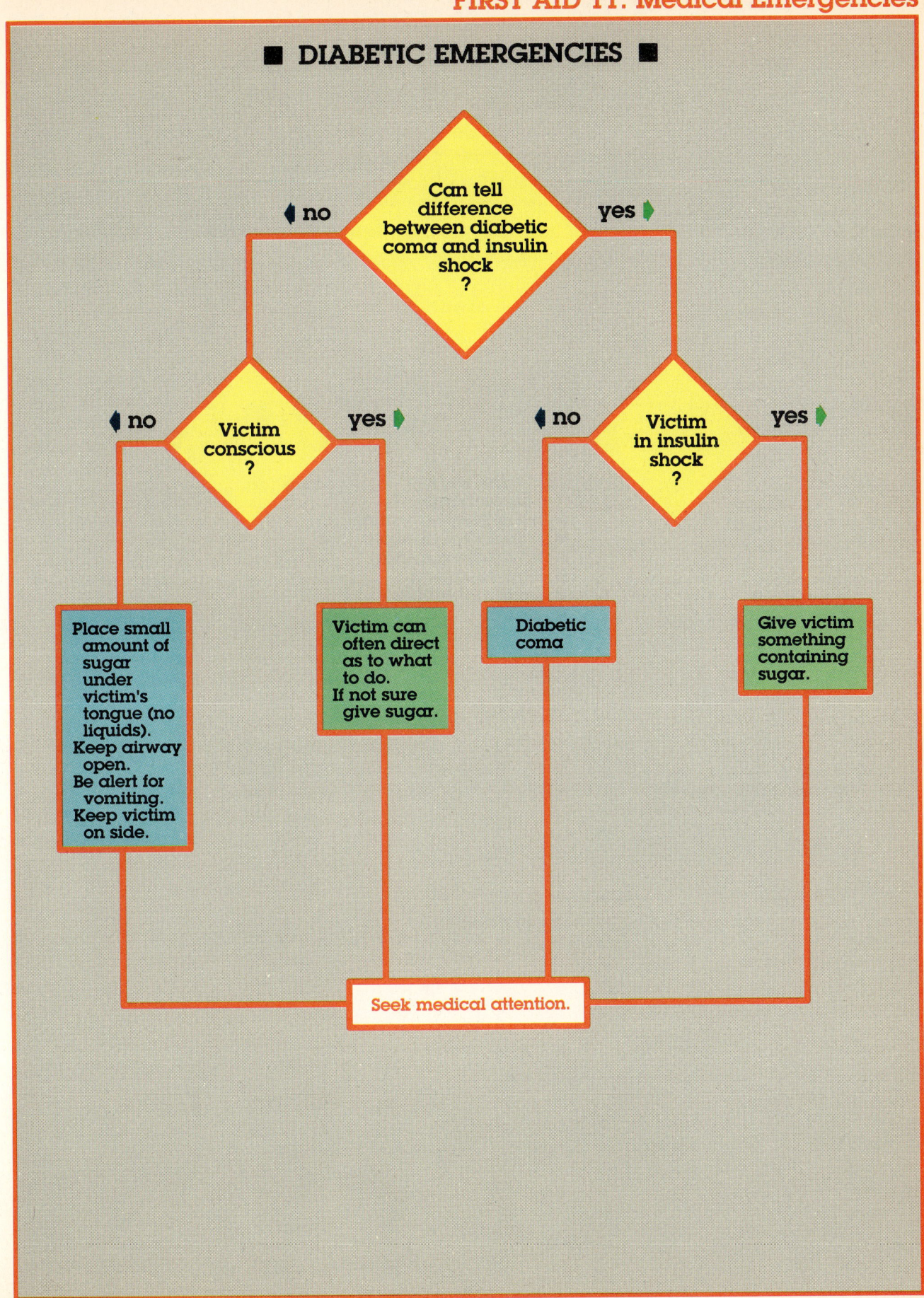

FIRST AID 11: Medical Emergencies

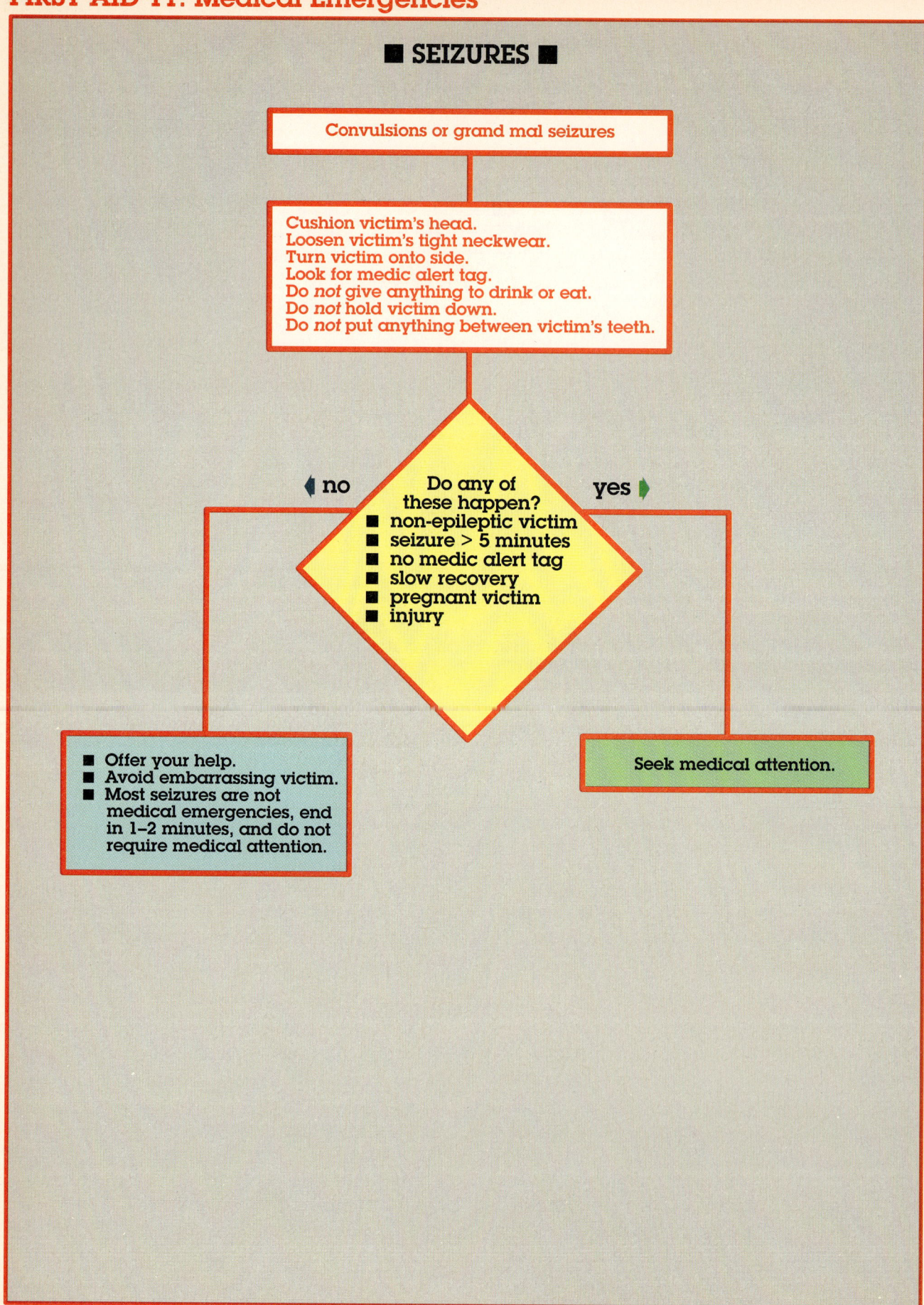

12
First Aid Skills

Dressings control bleeding and prevent contamination. Bandages hold dressings in place. Dressings come in many different forms. Sterile gauzes are most commonly used. When these cannot be found, nonsterile substances such as towels or handkerchiefs can be applied. Many different forms of bandages exist. Roller gauze, triangular, and cravat bandages make up the bandages most often used by first aiders. However, self-adhering and formfitting bandages have become popular especially with emergency medical technicians.

Bandages need not be textbook-perfect as long as they hold the dressings in place. Care should be taken, however, so that bandages are not applied too tightly or too loosely. Too tightly applied bandages will restrict blood flow, and too loose bandages fail to hold the dressing in place. When extremities are bandaged, the fingers and toes should be left exposed so that any color changes in them can be noted. Such changes may indicate impaired circulation. Pain, color change, numbness, and tingling represent other signs of a too-tight bandage.

Methods of applying dressings and bandages vary greatly and differ according to the types used and the injured part to which they are applied. Because of the variety of good bandaging techniques, the examples shown on the following pages represent a consensus among first aid experts as to the appropriate methods.

The following illustrations show suggested bandaging and splinting skills. This compilation represents the skills needed for first aid situations most likely to be encountered.

Suggested First Aid Kit Contents

Activated charcoal
Adhesive strip bandages, assorted sizes
Adhesive tape, 1- and 2-inch rolls
Alcohol (70%)
Alcohol wipes
Antimicrobial skin ointment (mycin family or triple antibiotic)
Baking soda
Calamine lotion
Chemical ice pack
Cotton balls
Cotton swabs
Decongestant tablets and spray
Diarrhea medication
Disposable gloves, latex
Elastic bandages, 2- and 3-inch widths
Extractor™ (Sawyer) if in snake country
Face mask with one-way valve
National Safety Council's First Aid Guide
Flashlight (small) and extra batteries
Gauze pads, 2 × 2 and 4 × 4 inches
Glutose™ (concentrated sugar)
Hot-water bottle
Household ammonia
Hydrocortisone cream (1%)
Hydrogen peroxide
Hypoallergenic tape
Ice bag (plastic)
Matches
Measuring cup and spoons

Moleskin
Needles
Non-adhering dressing
Oil of cloves
Over-the-counter pain medication (aspirin and acetaminophen)
Over-the-counter antihistamine
Paper and pencil
Paper drinking cups
Roller, self-adhering gauze, 2- to 4-inch widths
Rubber tubing
Safety pins, various sizes
Salt
Scissors
Soap
Space blanket
Spenco 2nd Skin™
Sam Splint™
Sugar
Sunscreen
Syrup of ipecac
Thermometer—1 oral, 1 rectal
Triangular bandages, 2 or 3
Tweezers
Waterproof tape
Zinc oxide

These items can be placed in a fishing tackle box for storage and transporting.

SKILL SCAN: Bandaging—Roller, Figure-of-Eight (Self-adhering)

ROLLER BANDAGE FOR HAND

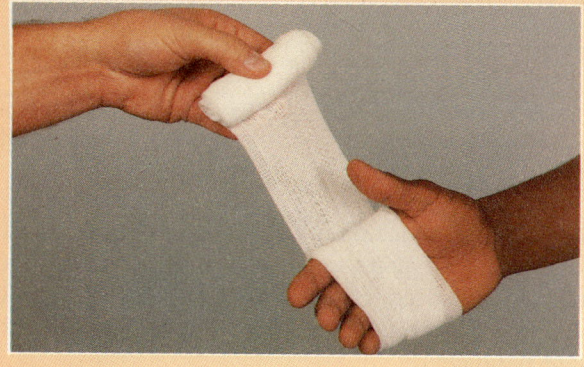

1.

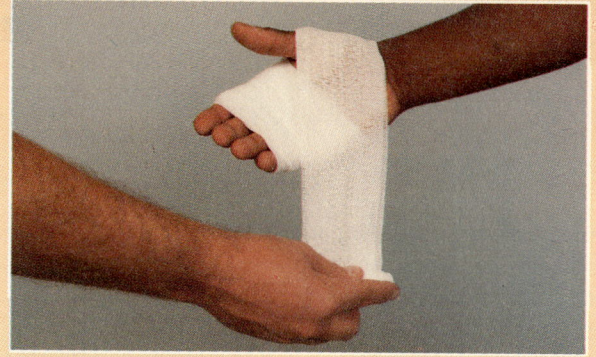

2.

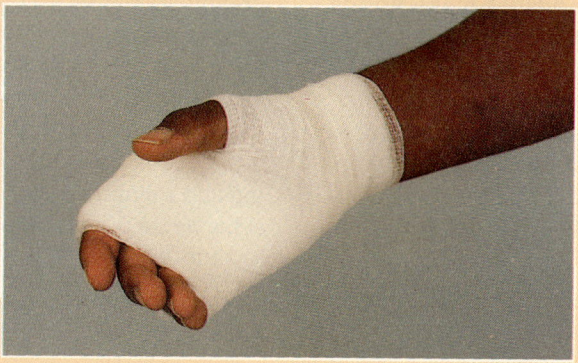

3.

ROLLER BANDAGE FOR ANKLE

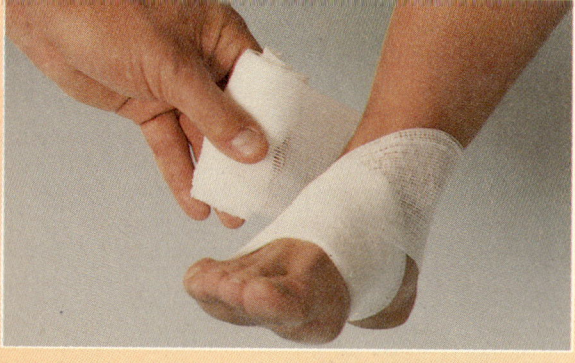

1.

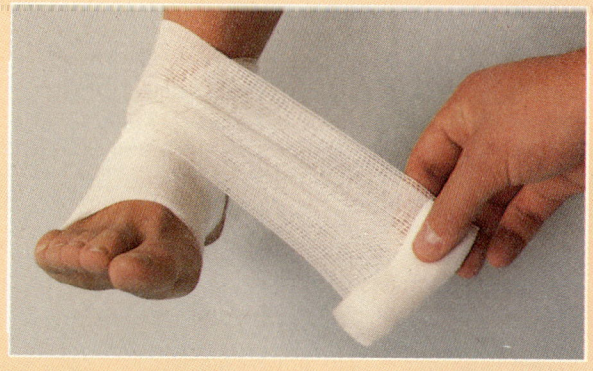

2.

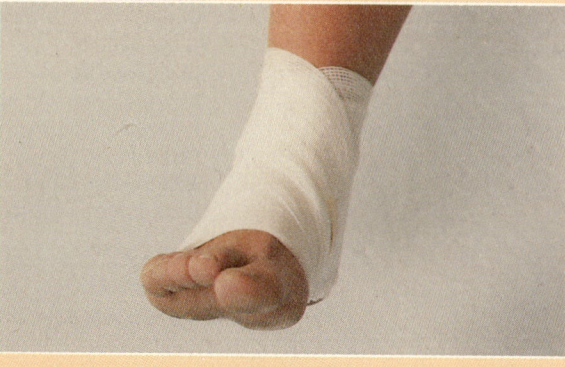

3.

SKILL SCAN: Splinting—Upper Extremities

ARM SLING: COLLARBONE, SHOULDER

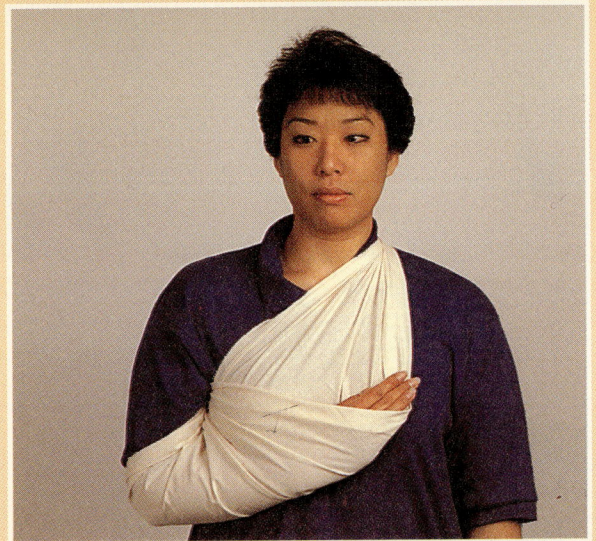

1.

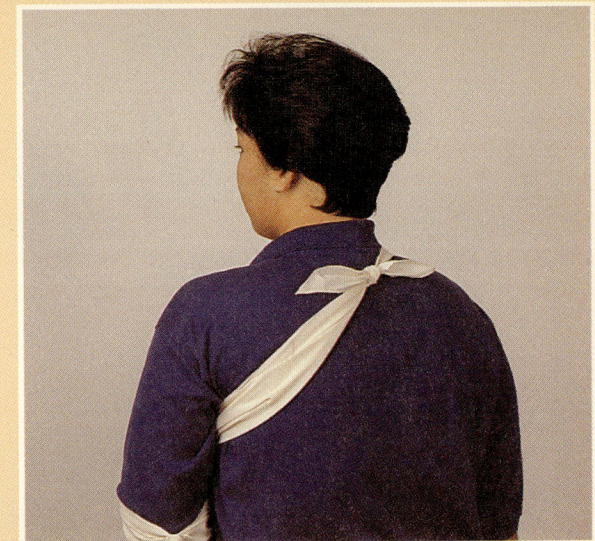

2.

ARM SLING AND SWATH (BINDER)

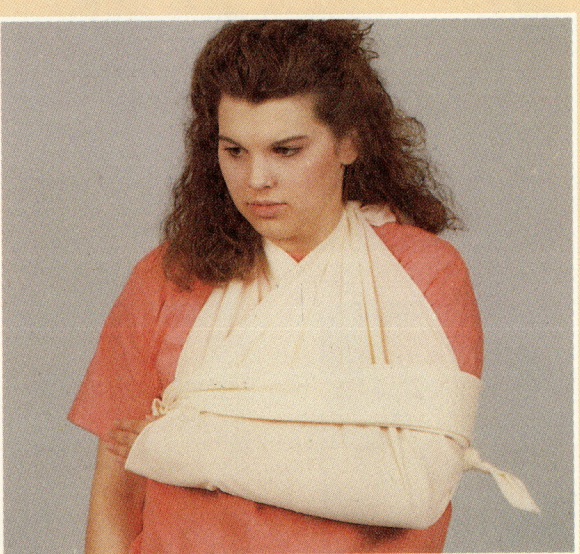

3.

FOREARM (RADIUS/ULNA)

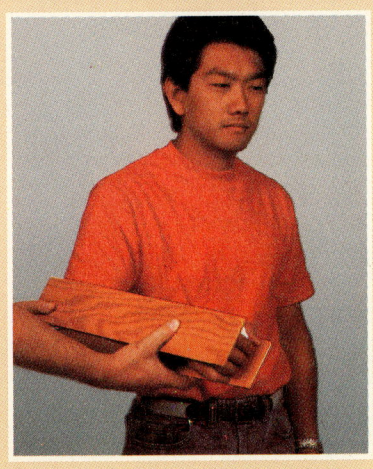

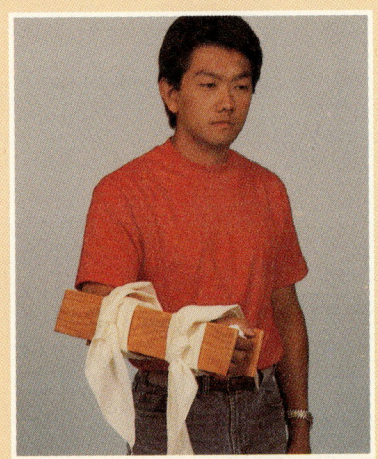

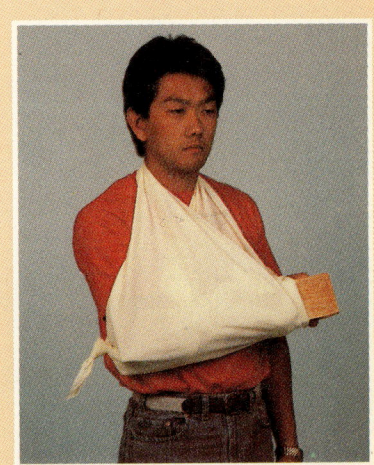

SKILL SCAN: Splinting—Lower Extremities

SPLINTING THE LOWER LEG (TIBIA/FIBULA)

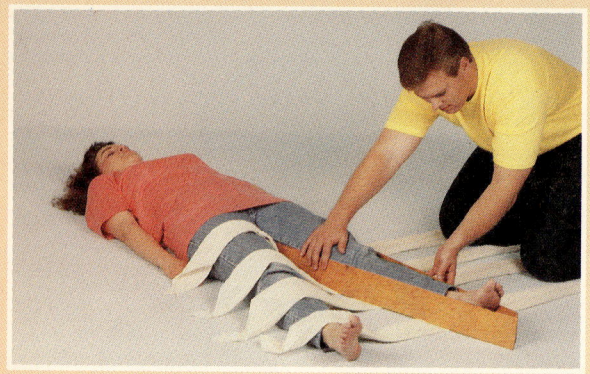
1.

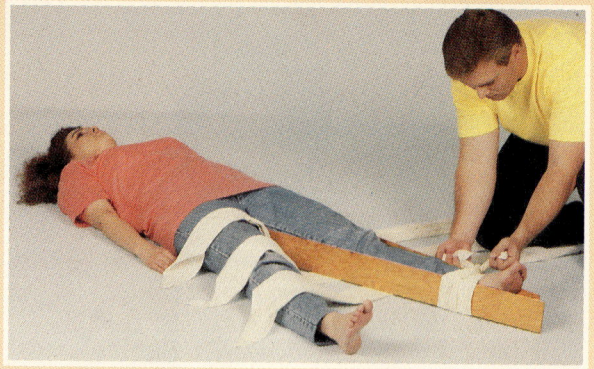
2.

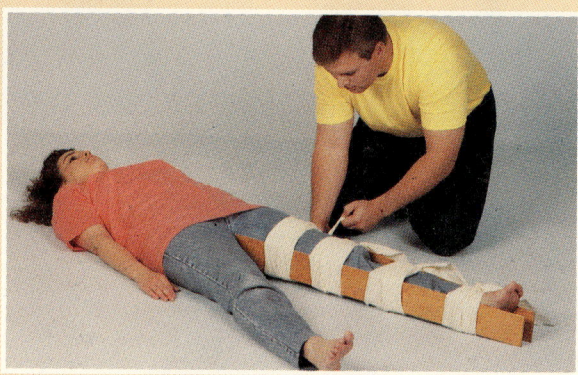
3.

THIGH (FEMUR)

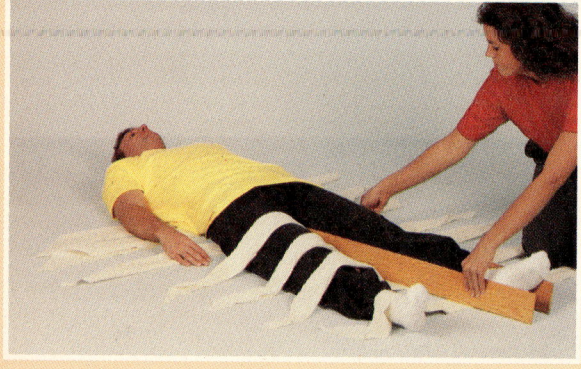
1.

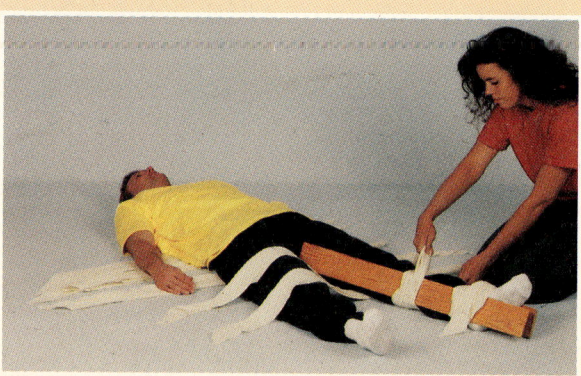
2.

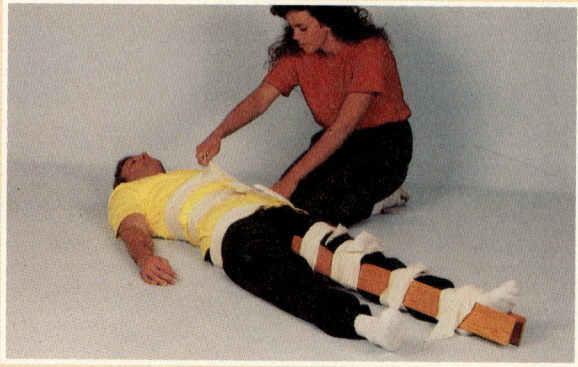
3.

SKILL SCAN: Splinting—Lower Extremities

ANKLE/FOOT

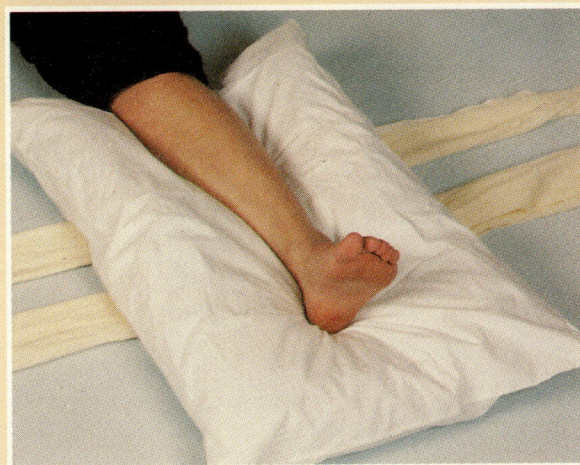

1.

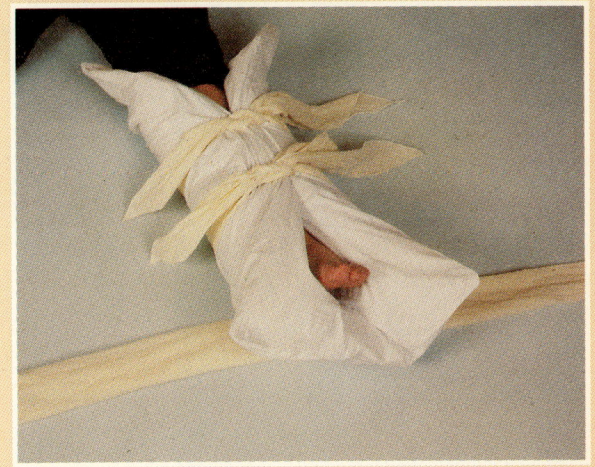

2.

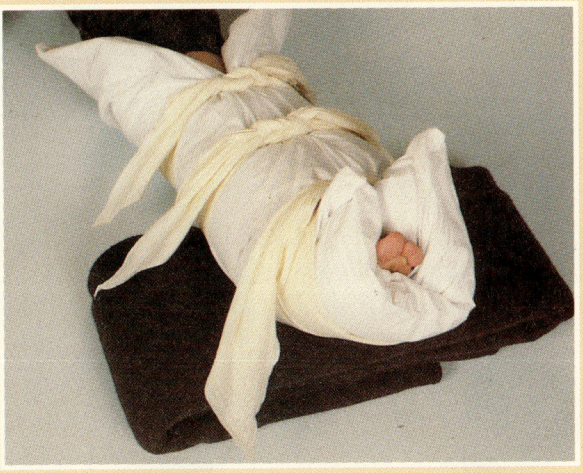

3.

SPLINTING—SELF-SPLINT

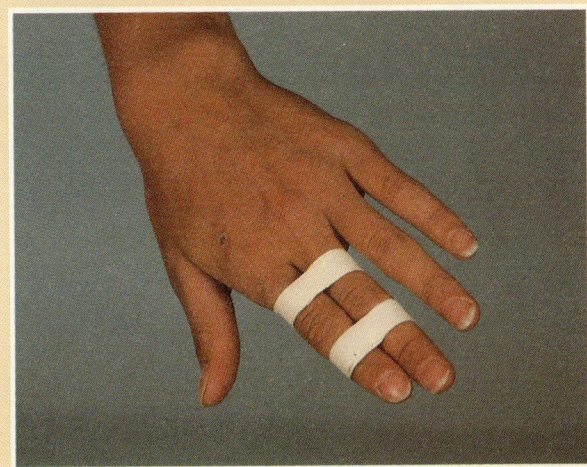

Fingers/toes

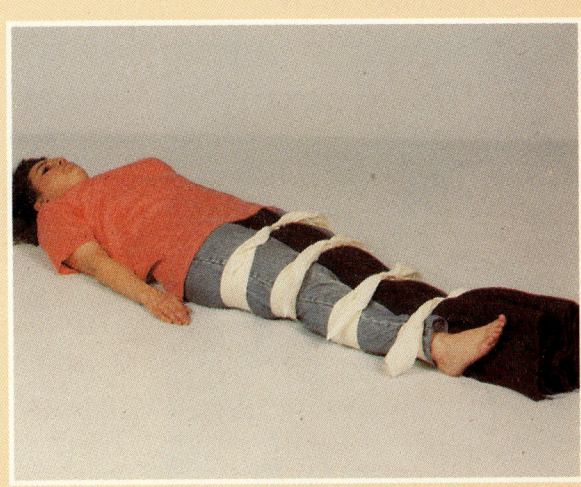

Leg

SKILL SCAN: Emergency Moves

ONE-PERSON MOVES

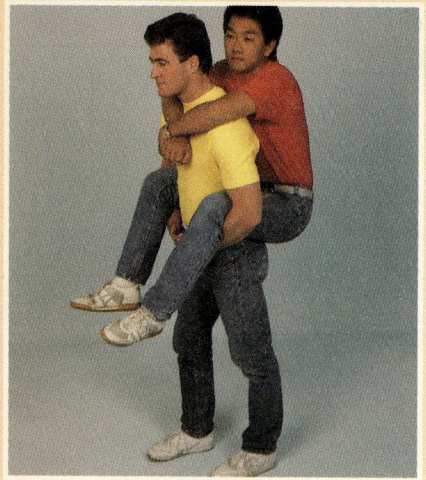

Piggyback carry

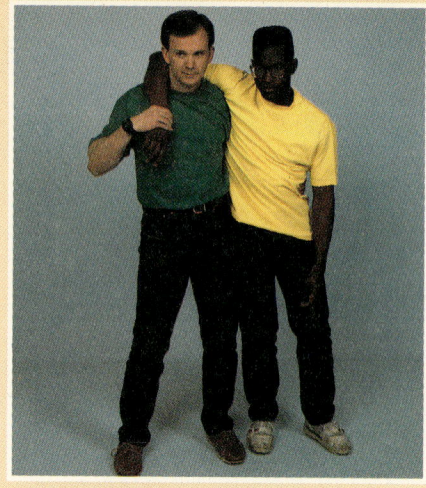

One-person assist

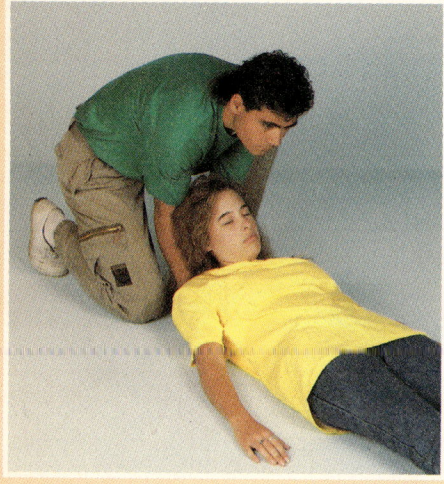

Shoulder drag

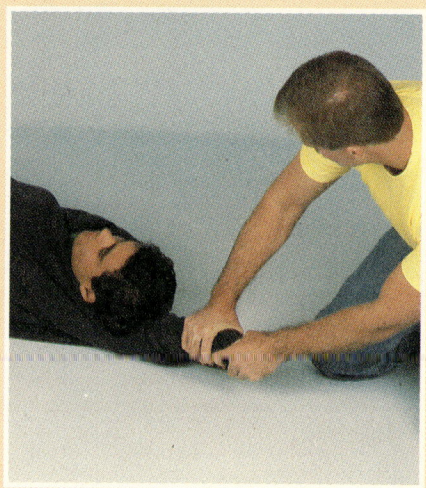

Blanket drag

TWO-PERSON MOVES

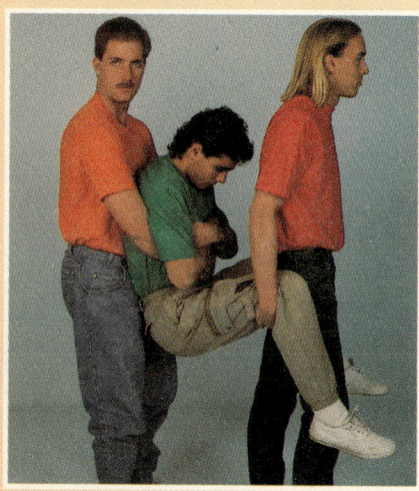

Extremity carry

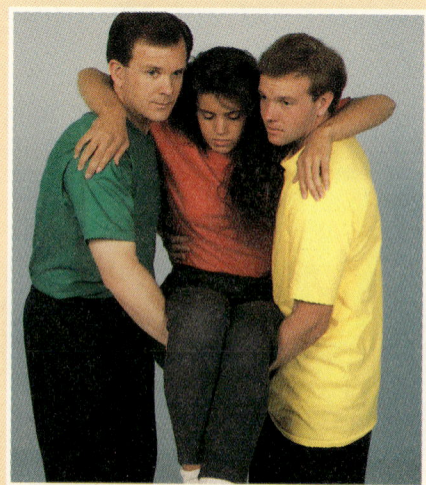

Two-handed seat carry

13
Moving and Rescuing Victims

In general, a victim should not be moved until he or she is ready for transportation to a hospital, if required. All necessary first aid should be provided first. A victim should be moved only if there is an immediate danger to him or others if he is not moved, that is:

- There is a fire or danger of fire.
- Explosives or other hazardous materials are involved.
- It is impossible to protect the accident scene.
- It is impossible to gain access to other victims in a vehicle who need life-saving care.

Note that a cardiac arrest victim would typically be moved unless he or she were on the ground or floor because cardiopulmonary resuscitation must be performed on a firm surface.

If it is necessary to move a victim, the speed with which he is moved depends on the reason for moving him, for example:

- **Emergency move.** If there is a fire, pull the victim away from the area as quickly as possible.
- **Nonemergency move.** If the victim needs to be moved to gain access to others in a vehicle, give due consideration to his injuries before and during movement.

Emergency Moves

The major danger in moving a victim quickly is the possibility of aggravating spine injury. In an emergency, every effort should be made to pull the victim in the direction of the long axis of the body to provide as much protection to the spine as possible. If the victim is on the floor or ground, you can drag her away from the scene by tugging on her clothing in the neck and shoulder area. It may be easier to pull the victim onto a blanket and then drag the blanket away from the scene. Such moves are emergency moves only. They do not adequately protect the spine from further injury.

Nonemergency Moves

All injured parts should be immobilized before moving and then protected during the moving. To protect yourself, you should use the following principles in all nonemergency moves:

- Keep in mind physical capabilities and limitations and do not try to handle too heavy a load. When in doubt, seek help.
- Keep yourself balanced when carrying out the move.
- Maintain a firm footing.
- Maintain a constant and firm grip.
- Lift and lower by bending your legs and not your back—keep your back as straight as possible at all times; bend knees and lift with one foot ahead of the other.
- When holding or transporting, keep your back straight and rely on shoulder and leg muscles; tighten muscles of your abdomen and buttocks.
- When performing a task that requires pulling, keep your back straight and pull using your arms and shoulders.
- Carry out all tasks slowly, smoothly, and in unison with your partner.
- Move your body gradually; avoid twisting and jerking when conducting the various victim-handling tasks.
- When handling a victim, try to keep your arms as close as possible to the body in order to maintain balance.
- Do not keep your muscles contracted for a long period of time.

Water Rescue

About 7,000 Americans die each year from drowning, making it the third leading cause of accidental death. Drowning statistics do not reflect the whole problem. An estimated 70,000 people are near-drowning victims each year. Even this figure does not give the entire picture because in many instances the victim recovers and the incident is not reported.

Since drowning situations seem to happen all the time, especially during the summer months, all adults and teenagers should be familiar with the basic rescue techniques available to poor swimmers or nonswimmers.

Reach-Throw-Row-Go

Reach-throw-row-go identifies the priority list for attempting a rescue.

Reach

The first and simplist rescue technique is the reach. This method is easily mastered, but it requires the ability to judge distance accurately and a lightweight pole, ladder, long stick, or any object that can be extended to the victim.

Once you have your "reacher," secure your footing. Also have a bystander grab your belt or pants for stability. Make sure you are secure before reaching down to assist the victim. Keep talking; this not only calms the victim, it helps you think through each step.

Throw

Throwing is another elementary rescue. It provides a maximum range of about fifty feet for the average untrained rescuer. You can throw anything that floats—objects such as empty fuel or paint cans, plastic containers, life jackets or floating cushions, short pieces of wood—whatever is available. If there is rope handy, tie it to the object to be thrown because you can retrieve it in case you miss.

Row

If the victim is beyond reach and you can find a nearby sailboard, boogie board, rowboat, canoe, or an outboard craft that can be started, you may attempt this form of rescue. Using these crafts requires skill only acquired through practice. In a life-or-death situation, however, even the inept use of these craft will be safer and faster than a swimming rescue. There is an element of danger for the rescuer that should be considered.

Craft powered by hand, paddle, or oar may be slower, but they are safer than a motor-driven craft with which you are unfamiliar. Inexperienced hands on a throttle are more dangerous than inexperienced hands on an oar.

If rowing out to a victim, align with an object on the shoreline and in line with the victim. Fix this in your memory. Since you must row facing the opposite direction, you will need to turn your head every five or so strokes to check on the victim and your position.

Upon reaching the victim, never attempt to pull the victim in over the sides of a boat but over the stern, or rear end. The former method has been the cause of countless double drownings.

Go

If the previous "reach-throw-row" priorities are impossible to do, you must make an assessment, weighing the potential risk to yourself versus the reward to the victim. Entering even calm water to make a swimming rescue is difficult and hazardous. It takes skill, training, and excellent physical condition. All too frequently a would-be rescuer becomes a victim as well.

After the Rescue

Once the victim is out of the water, protect yourself and the victim against the cold. Get into dry clothing as soon as possible. Be prepared to administer mouth-to-mouth or CPR resuscitation. All rescued victims should be seen by a physician and hospitalized because victims can die a few minutes or up to 96 hours after the incident of secondary complications. Aspiration pneumonia is a late complication of near-drowning episodes, occurring after 48 to 72 hours have elapsed.

Ice Rescue

Attempt to reach the person from shore with a long object (e.g., a branch, a rope, or a board). If there is no equipment, form a human chain reaching from the shore. Lie flat to distribute the weight. Seek medical attention immediately for someone who has fallen through broken ice.

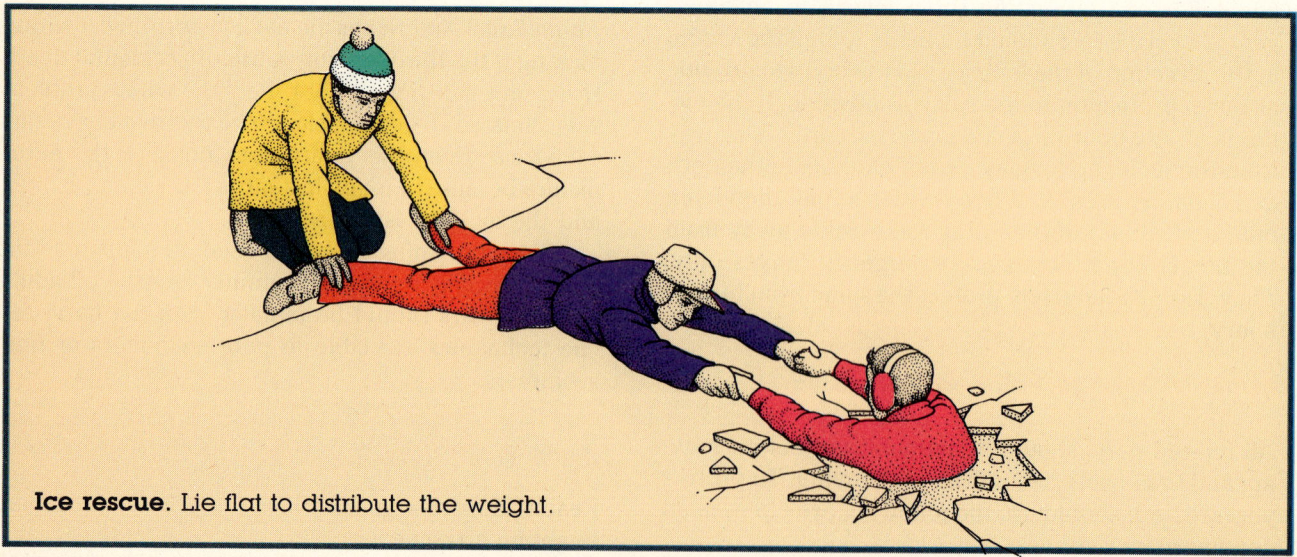

Ice rescue. Lie flat to distribute the weight.

SKILL SCAN: Water Rescue

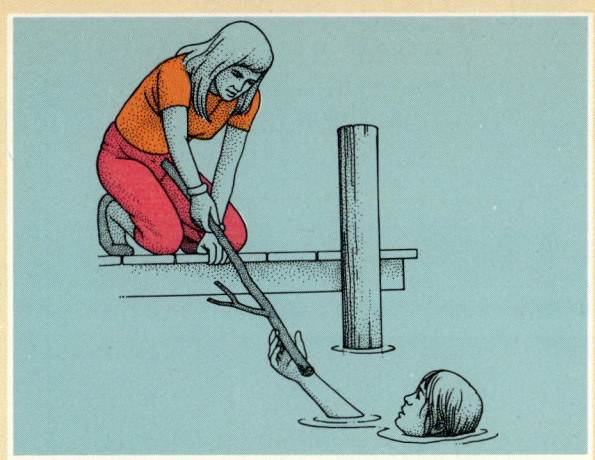

1. Reach the person from shore.

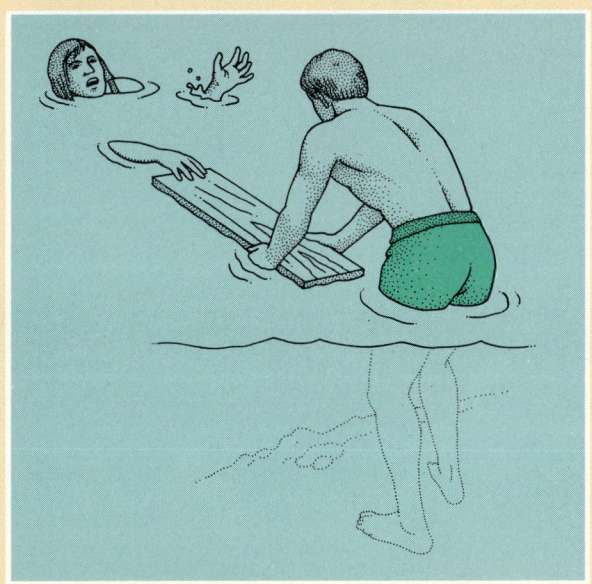

2. If you cannot reach the person from shore, wade closer.

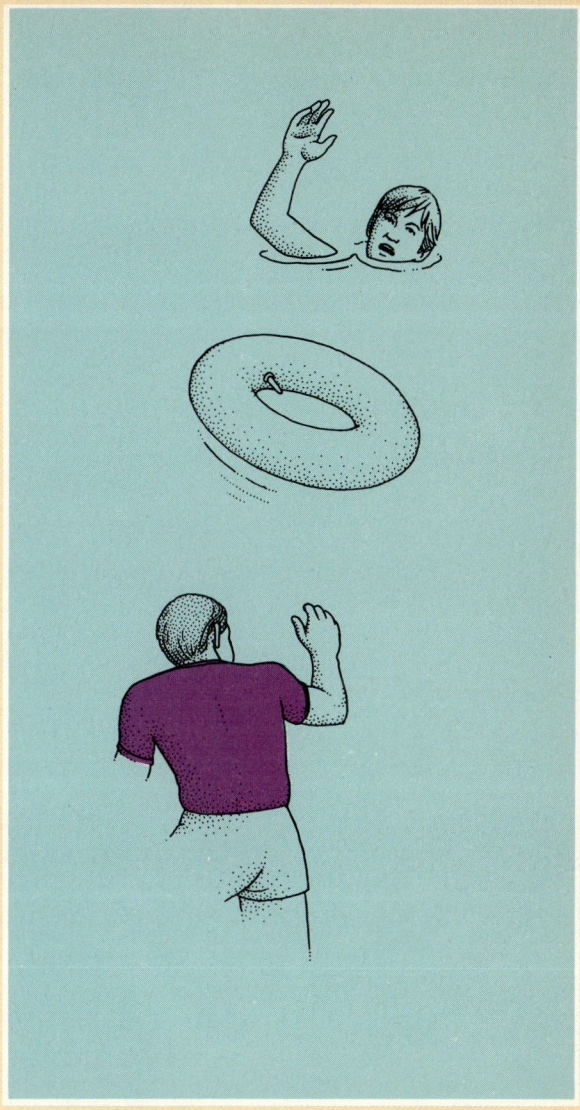

3. If an object that floats is available, throw it to the person.

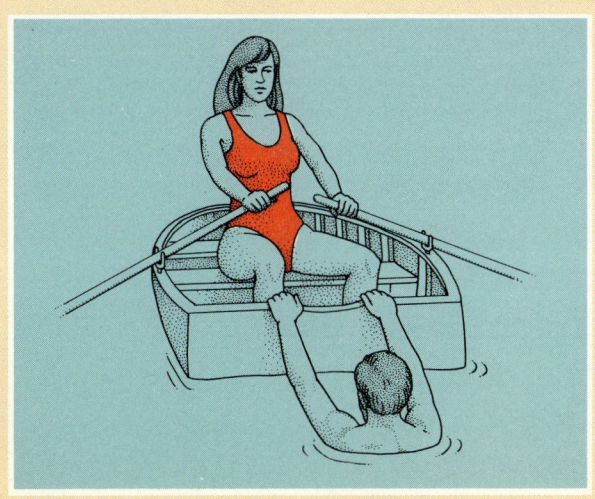

4. Use a boat if one is available.

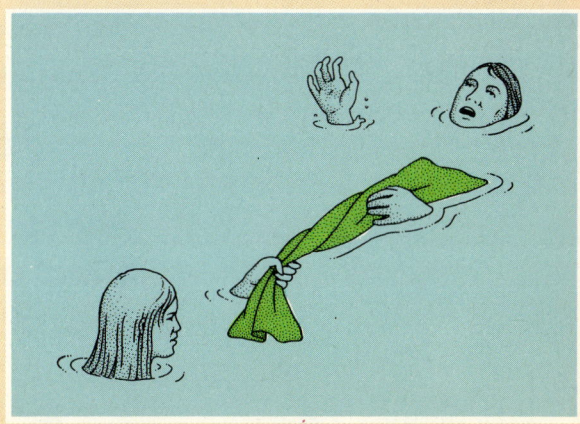

5. If you must swim to the person, use a towel or board for him or her to hold onto. Do not let the person grab you.

Quick Emergency Index

Abdominal injuries, 45
Bleeding, 33
Blisters, 46
Chemical burns, 63
Chest injuries, 44
Dental injuries, 43
Diabetic emergencies, 81
Electrical injuries, 64
Eye injuries, 41
Fainting, 28
Fractures, 73
Frostbite, 68
Head injuries, 40
Heart attack, 79
Heat burns, 62
Heat-related emergencies, 70
Hypothermia, 69
Hypovolemic shock, 27
Inhaled poison, 57
Insect stings, 52
Muscle injuries, 75
Nosebleeds, 42
Poison ivy, 56
Seizures, 82
Severe allergic reaction, 29
Snakebites, 53
Spinal injuries, 74
Spider bites and scorpion stings, 54
Sprains, strains, contusions, dislocations, 76
Stroke, 80
Swallowed poison, 51
Tick removal, 55